Lupus - Need to Know

Edited by Reem Hamdy A. Mohammed

Published in London, United Kingdom

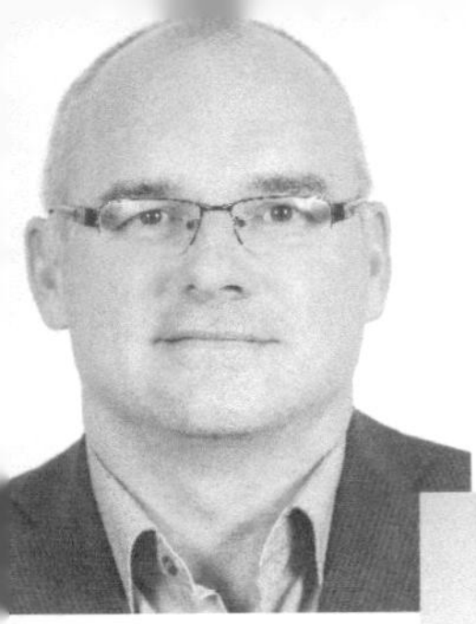
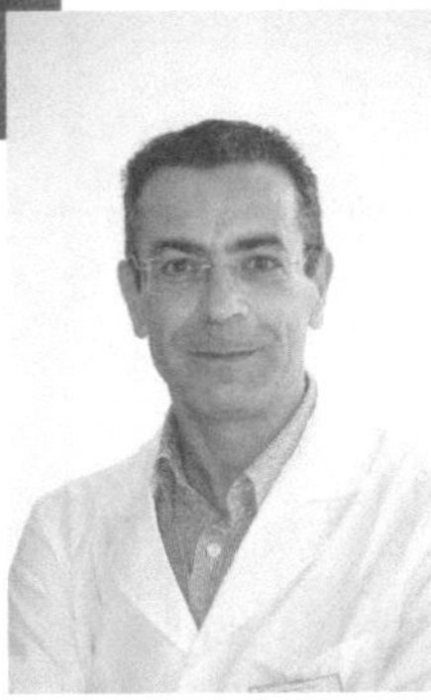
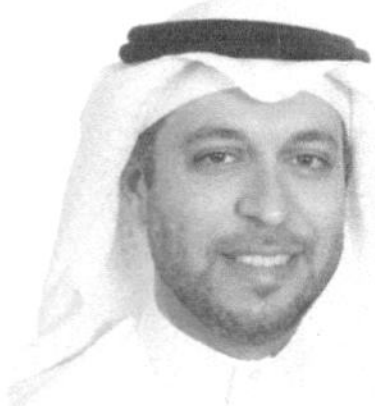
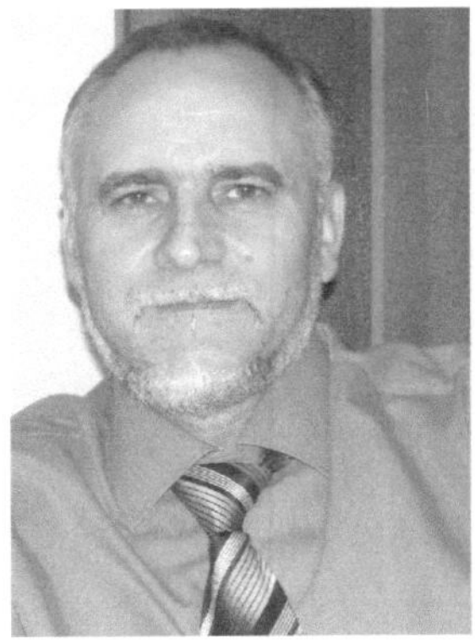
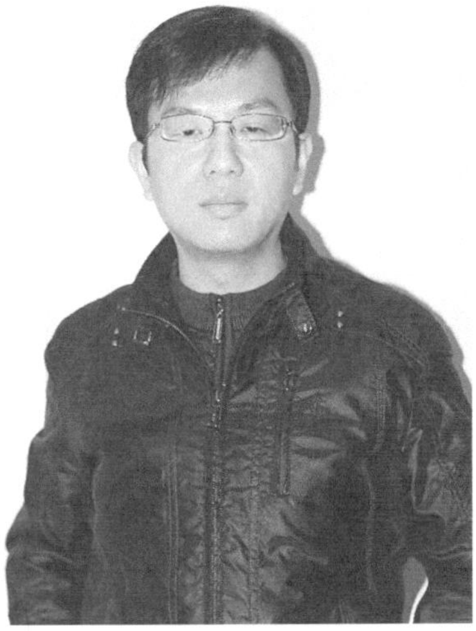
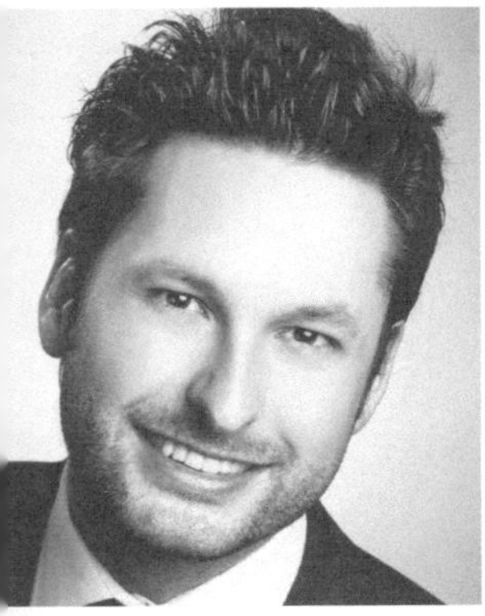
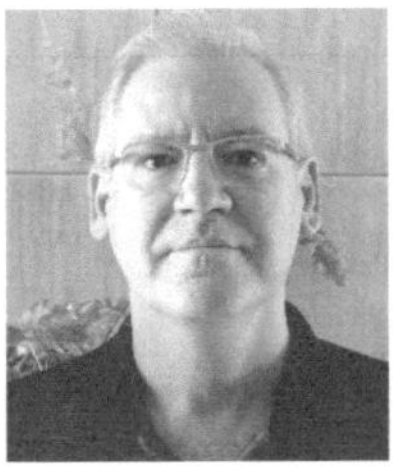

IntechOpen

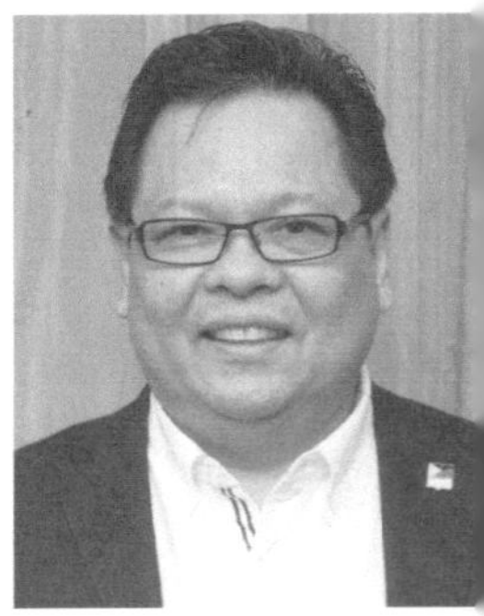
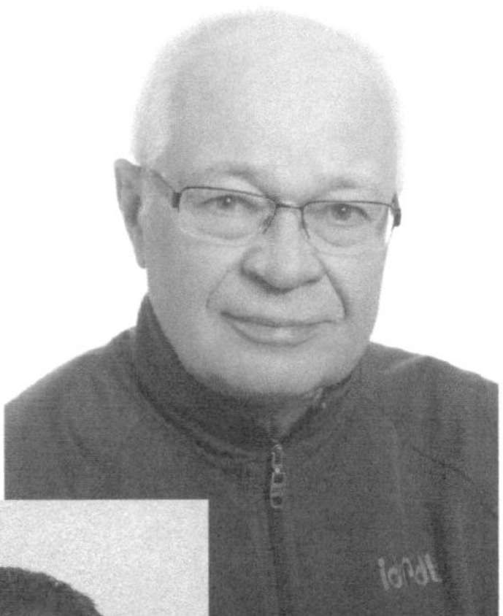
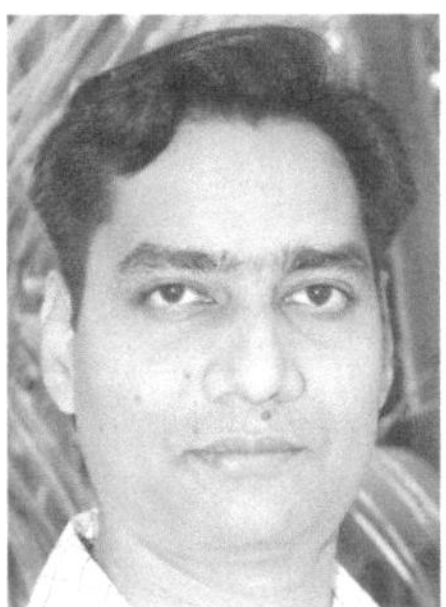
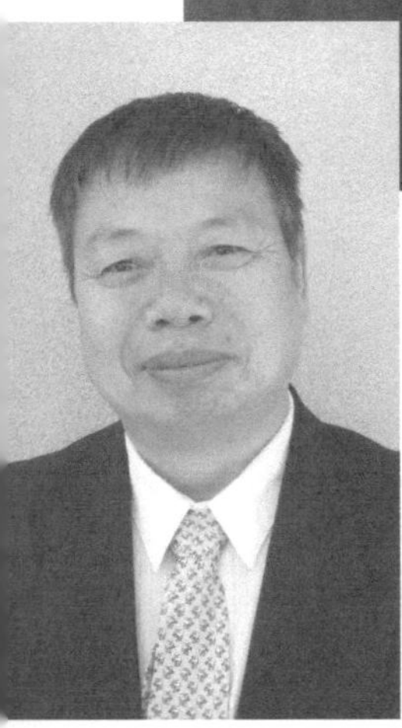
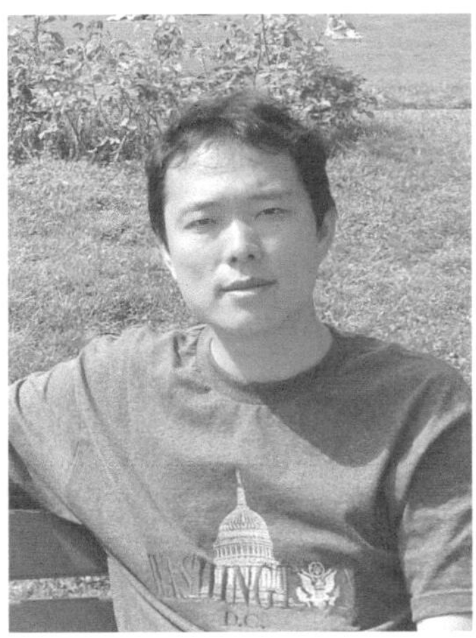
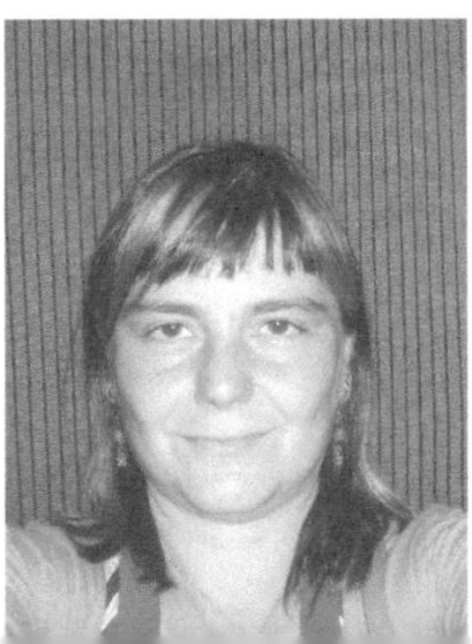

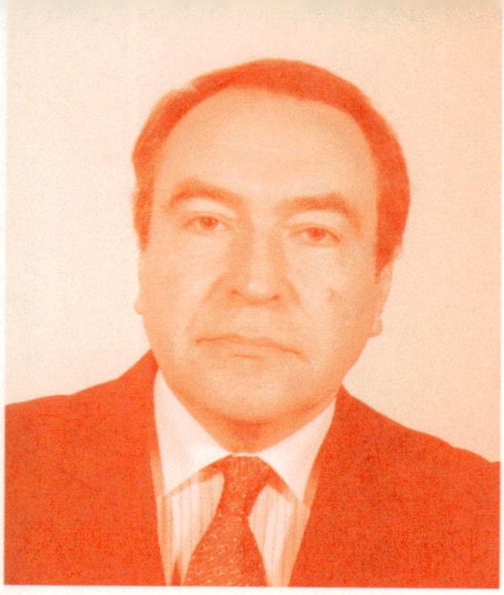
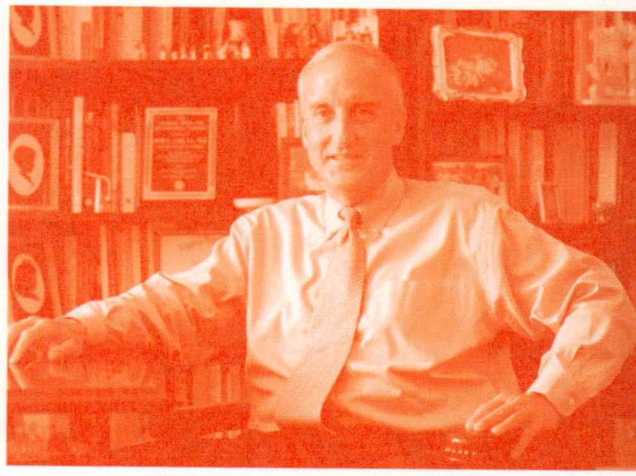
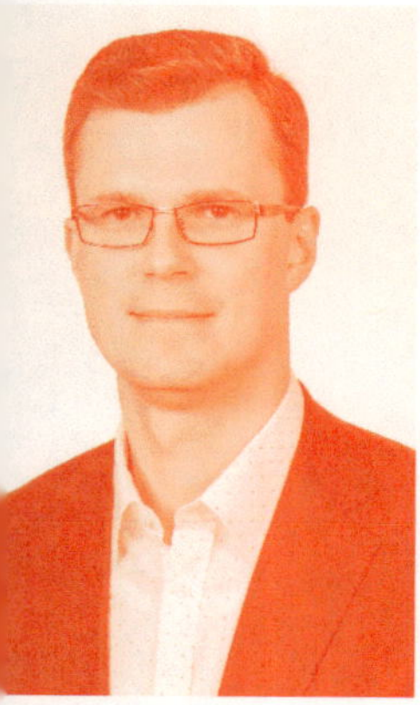
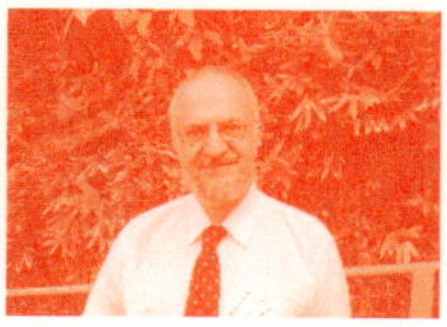
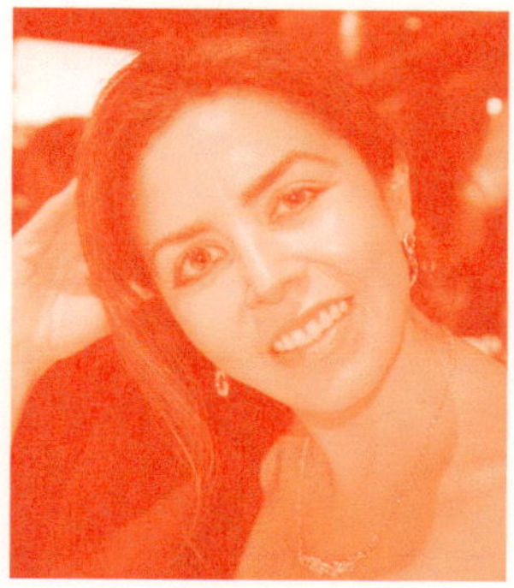

Supporting open minds since 2005

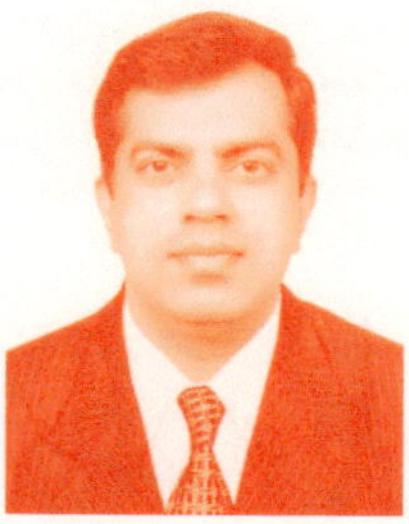
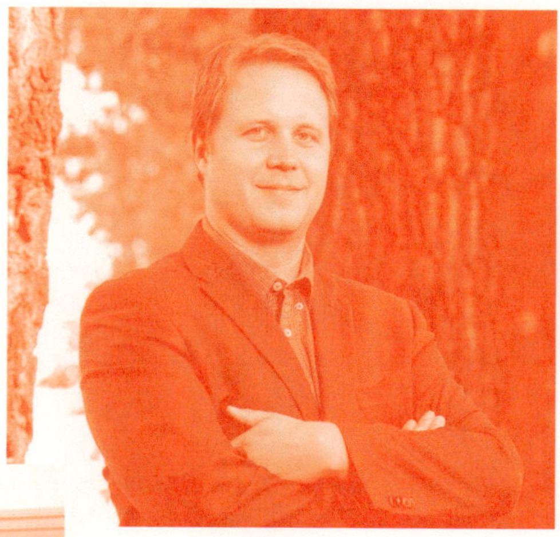
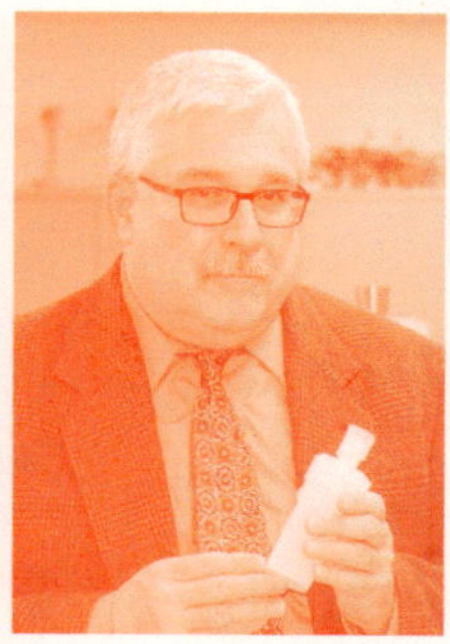
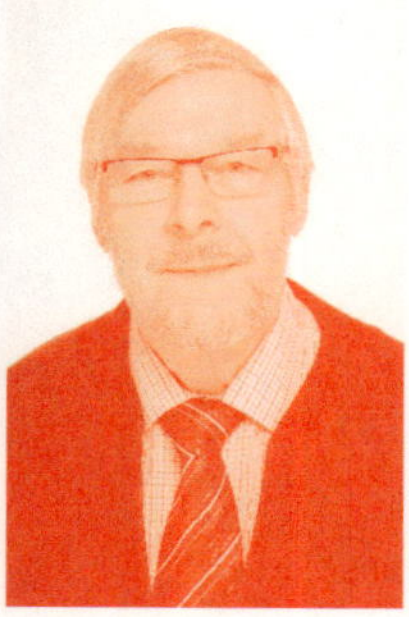
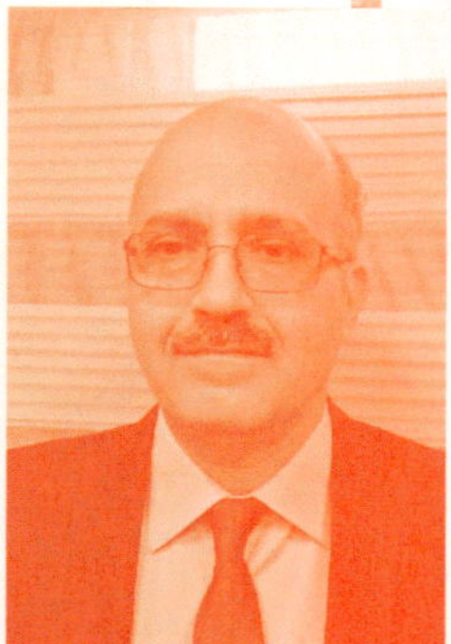
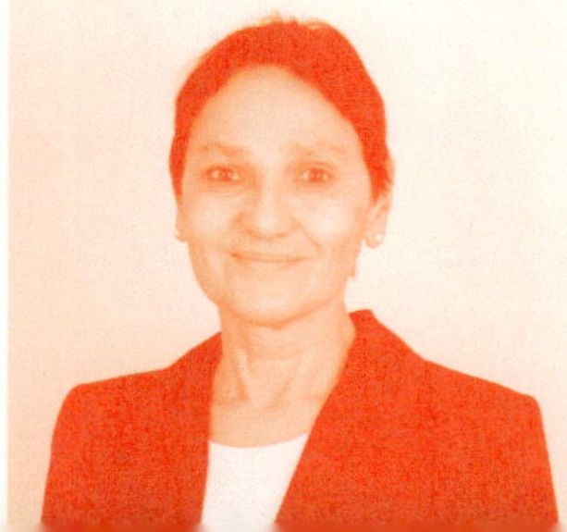
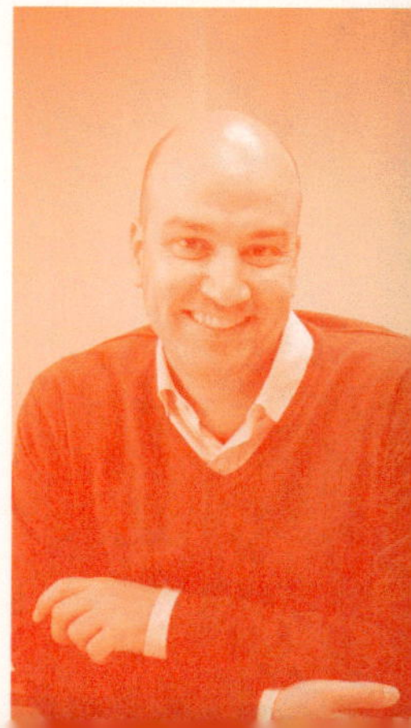

Lupus - Need to Know
http://dx.doi.org/10.5772/intechopen.83100
Edited by Reem Hamdy A. Mohammed

Part of IntechOpen Book Series: Rheumatology, Volume 5
Book Series Editor: Maria Maślińska

Contributors
Ifigenia Kostoglou-Athanassiou, Panagiotis Athanassiou, Lambros Athanassiou, Rosa Marlene Viero, Daniela Cristina dos Santos, Gurinder Kumar, Hulya Bukulmez, Stephen Soloway, Fahd Adeeb, Wan Ahmad Hafiz Wan Md Adnan, Vera Bernardino, Melissa Fernandes, Anna Taulaigo, Ana Lladó, Jorge Fernandes, Fátima Serrano

First published in London, United Kingdom, 2021 by IntechOpen
IntechOpen is the global imprint of INTECHOPEN LIMITED, registered in England and Wales, registration number: 11086078, 5 Princes Gate Court, London, SW7 2QJ, United Kingdom
Printed in Croatia

British Library Cataloguing-in-Publication Data
A catalogue record for this book is available from the British Library

Additional hard and PDF copies can be obtained from orders@intechopen.com

Lupus - Need to Know
Edited by Reem Hamdy A. Mohammed
p. cm.
Print ISBN 978-1-83968-403-6
Online ISBN 978-1-83968-405-0
eBook (PDF) ISBN 978-1-83968-406-7
ISSN 2631-9233

IntechOpen Book Series
Rheumatology
Volume 5

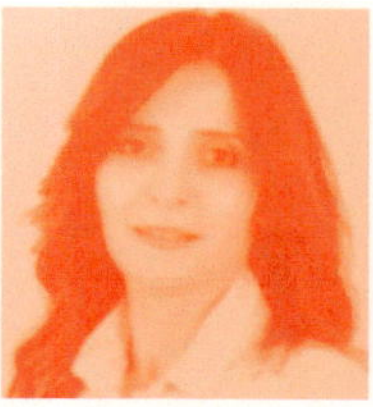

Professor Reem Hamdy Abdellatif Mohammed graduated from the School of Medicine, Cairo University, Egypt, where she is currently a Professor of Rheumatology and Clinical Immunology. She is a fellow of the Royal College of Physicians and a Certified International Professional Trainer (CIPT) at the Faculty and Leadership Development Center (FLDC), Cairo University, and at the Management Development Institute, Missouri State University, USA, carrying on teaching and training on the “Establishment of the Evidence-Based Strategy in Medical Research and Practice.” Dr. Mohammed is a verified editor, reviewer, and advisory board member for several reputable international journals. She is also a member of the “Capacity Building Team” at Cairo University. She is the author and co-author of several books and an international speaker in the field of rheumatology and immunology.
Scopus Author ID: 35280107100 ORCID ID: ORCID logohttps://orcid.org/0000-0003-4994-7687 CU Scholar account: https://scholar.cu.edu.eg/?q=reemhamdy/publications

Editor of Volume 5:
Reem Hamdy Abdellatif Mohammed
Professor of Rheumatology and Clinical Immunology-
Department of Rheumatology and rehabilitation-
School of Medicine- Cairo University.
Cairo -Egypt

Book Series Editor:
Maria Maślińska
National Institute of Geriatrics, Rheumatology and Rehabilitation
Early Arthritis Clinic, Warsaw, Poland

Scope of the Series

This book series presents new concepts of pathogenesis, including genetic, epigenetic determinants and epidemiology of rheumatic diseases. It focuses on current classification criteria, recommendations for the diagnosis and treatment of rheumatic diseases. The goal of the series is to explain various aspects of disorders associated with impaired immune response and autoimmunity processes. It also discusses risk factors associated with the development of autoimmune diseases, as well as latest discoveries and future perspectives of this extremely dynamic field of internal medicine - rheumatology.

Contents

Preface

Systemic lupus erythematosus (SLE) is a multisystem, immune-mediated, inflammatory disease of unknown etiology. Lupus has always featured a broad spectrum of disease-related manifestations that pose significant challenges to successful intervention.

This book presents scientific updates in specific clinical situations to provide meaningful insight into effective control strategies for SLE in rheumatology practice. Chapter authors provide comprehensive information on difficult-to-treat disease-related problems and their evidence-based lines of management. The book begins with a brief guide to diagnosing disease with a vast array of heterogeneous manifestations and mimics. The next section provides an update on lupus kidney disease. Considering the frequency and burden of lupus renal disease, the authors provide a full section on updates in the diagnosis and therapy of lupus nephritis. The next section focuses on endocrinopathies in lupus followed by a section on lupus and pregnancy. The final section examines advances in disease-targeted therapy as well as current and future perspectives.

To my husband Hesham, daughter Maya, and son Karim, who have always inspired and encouraged me not to give up on my dreams.

Reem Hamdy A. Mohammed
Professor of Rheumatology and Clinical Immunology,
Department of Rheumatology and Rehabilitation,
School of Medicine,
Cairo University,
Cairo, Egypt

Section 1

Systemic Lupus Erythematosus: Pick the Case

Chapter 1

Don't Miss Lupus

Stephen Soloway

Abstract

Chapter for Lupus Book Systemic lupus erythematosus is a well-recognized multi-system disease. Hallmarks of the disorder include the prevalence of anti-nuclear antibodies (ANA) and double stranded antibodies (DNA). The disease often presents with lupus rashes and/or arthritis or arthralgias. Lupus is "the great imitator," as no organ system is excluded, when diagnosing and treating a lupus patient. While lupus remains evasive in novel therapies with true benefit; one issue has been consistent, in that the preponderance of the evidence thus far, leads to B cell dysfunction. More recently Belimumab was indicated for use in lupus patients. This is a BLyS-Specific inhibitor (B lymphocyte stimulator) medication. At this time, I would like to focus on lupus in a manner that you are not used to hearing. Typically, any practitioner who approaches a patient with a plethora of symptoms, would order blood tests, and conclude a diagnosis of lupus. In this chapter, I will point out and focus on the need to think "outside the box" and perhaps consider lupus as simply one of various other scenarios.

Keywords: lupus, Sjogren's, Raynaud's, ANA, DNA, DRV VT

1. Introduction

1.1 Hallmarks of systemic lupus erythematosus

Systemic lupus erythematosus is a well-recognized multi-system disease [1].

Hallmarks of the disorder include the prevalence of antinuclear antibodies (ANA) and double stranded antibodies (DNA). The disease often presents with rashes and/or arthritis or arthralgias. Lupus is "the great imitator," as no organ system is excluded, when diagnosing and treating a lupus patient.

1.2 Most recent development for lupus treatment

While lupus remains evasive in novel therapies with true benefit; one issue has been consistent, in that the preponderance of the evidence thus far, leads to B cell dysfunction. More recently Belimumab was indicated for use in lupus patients, which is an immunomodulator B-Lymphocyte Stimulator (BLyS)-Specific Inhibitor. This drug was approved by the Food and Drug Administration (FDA) for use in lupus patients in 2011 [2]. The majority of patients afflicted with lupus, autoreactive B-cells remain in the body longer than necessary. Belimumab binds to BLyS, causing it to no longer bind to and stimulate the autoreactive B cell.

Information recently discussed at the ACR2020, provides evidence of Belimumab standard therapy ameliorating the outcome for patients with active renal lupus. A combination of Belimumab, with either mycophenolate mofetil or

Azathioprine, was shown to be more effective than either of these therapies alone. While studies are not yet conclusive, a combination of Belimumab with cyclophosphamide, posed no higher risk than cyclophosphamide alone. This combination in a class IV nephritis group exceeded those who received cyclophosphamide alone [3].

Anifrolumab, an interleukin-1 inhibitor, was not shown to be effective in systemic lupus, it did show promise in TULIP-1 and 2 and skin lesions related to lupus. Anifrolumab's effect on non-skin lupus disease activity however, was nominal [4].

2. A rheum with a different view

In this section, lupus will be discussed pragmatically. Most practitioners are unaccustomed to viewing disease features from a rheumatologic standpoint. Typically, the practitioner that approaches a patient with a plethora of symptoms, would order blood tests, and conclude a diagnosis of lupus; however, in this part of the chapter, we will discuss the need to focus "outside the box" and perhaps consider lupus as simply one of various other scenarios.

2.1 Finding evidence of lupus

Features of lupus considered in the differential diagnoses of other conditions include rashes, arthritis, renal disease (glomerular or tubular), Raynaud's phenomenon, sicca syndrome and muscle weakness. The differential diagnoses for these features often include lymphoma, sarcoidosis, phospholipid antibody syndrome, rheumatoid arthritis, inflammatory myopathy, Sjogren's syndrome, IgG4-related disease and scleroderma.

A lupus rash, seen with or without vasculitis, typically small vessel-showing leukocytoclastic vasculitis, is seen at the dermal/epidermal junction with immunofluorescence positive for IgG and complements [5]. Small vessel vasculitis is responsible for much of the severe abdominal pain seen in lupus patients.

Arthritis of lupus is inflammatory but not erosive. Differential diagnoses would include rheumatoid arthritis, gout, or psoriatic arthritis. Rheumatoid arthritis, psoriatic arthritis, scleroderma, sarcoid and gout are all destructive arthritic diseases [6].

Renal pathology is often noted due to blood or protein in the urine. It may be diagnosed by a decrease in renal function, which is differentiated on biopsy. Lupus tends to involve glomerulus with a "full house" pattern on immunofluorescent staining (i.e., presence of glomerular deposits that stain for IgG, IgM, IgA, C3 and C1q). This is the only organ finding to satisfy the SLICC criteria on its own in patients with systemic lupus. IgG and complements would be suggestive of lupus nephritis in a patient with proliferative glomerulonephritis. This may be focal, diffuse or pure membranous nephropathy [7]. A patient with pure membranous disease, high double stranded DNA and low complements often do not apply. Proliferative lesions are often seen in the face of rising double stranded DNA and consumption of complement levels. These levels are not subject to change in Sjogren's, scleroderma, sarcoid, or IgG4-related disease. (IgG4-related disease is unique, as both tubulointerstitial diseases occur simultaneously with glomerular disease). ANCA vasculitis shows pauci-immune deposits [8], while sarcoidosis would show granulomas without positive stain for immunofluorescence. Goodpasture syndrome will show anti-GBM antibodies [9]. Sjogren's syndrome will show renal tubular acidosis, and only rarely, glomerular disease [10]. Most cases of tubulointerstitial nephritis are drug-induced, and may be caused by medications, such as antibiotics medications, NSAIDs, proton pump inhibitors, and immune-checkpoint inhibitors [11]. Uncommonly, NSAIDs may cause a combination of interstitial nephritis and nephrotic syndrome. Infections (i.e., legionella or *Mycobacterium tuberculosis* infection), may lead to a diagnosis of tubulointerstitial nephritis; however, autoimmune diseases, such as systemic lupus, sarcoidosis, Sjogren's syndrome, and uveitis syndrome, are also proven to cause tubulointerstitial nephritis [12]. Approximately 10–20% of patients diagnosed with lupus nephritis, have isolated lupus membranous nephropathy (class V), with no associated proliferative lesion present [13]. In patients with lupus nephritis, tubulointerstitial interstitial nephritis may accompany glomerular lesions, which is a risk factor for a poor outlook [14]. The IgG4 is a diagnostic differential and reveals tubulointerstitial nephritis, repeatedly associated with hypocomplementemia and hypodense nodular lesions, which can be seen on contrast-enhanced computerized tomography [15]. Tissue eosinophilia and deposits in the tubular basement membrane are often present, in addition to the distinctive pathological features of the disease [16].

Pulmonary renal syndromes can be seen in a very similar fashion, adding that lupus may present with acute glomerulonephritis, proliferative in nature, in addition to concurrent alveolar hemorrhage or diffuse interstitial infiltrates [17]. This pattern of disease seen in ANCA vasculitis is predominantly granulomatous polyangiitis, microscopic polyangiitis, and cryoglobulinemia, which is associated with hepatitis C infection [18].

Oral and ocular dryness, with or without uveitis, are features of lupus [19]. Uveitis is frequently seen in sarcoidosis and described in IgG4-related disease and HLA-B27-related conditions, while corneal-related disease has a differential diagnosis in rheumatoid arthritis, myopathy, and phospholipid antibody syndrome.

Primary muscle weakness while in lupus, [20] is part of a differential diagnoses that includes polymyositis, dermatomyositis, immune mediated necrotizing myopathy, lupus with myopathy, sarcoidosis with myopathy and Crohn's with myopathy. The latter two, show non-caseating granuloma disease on biopsy, while lupus shows diffuse immunofluorescence, mainly immunoglobulins and complements. This could be referred to as a "recurring theme" in lupus deposits of immunoglobulin and complements. Cocaine-laced with levamisole is in the differential diagnosis systemic lupus, myopathy and vasculitis [21].

A rheumatologist should recognize a lupus patient by the malar rash sparing the nasolabial folds, "classic kidney biopsy" and other constellations, such as "non-scarring alopecia" and "discoid lupus". These cases are often straightforward, and do not require biopsy. The classic malar rash sparing the nasolabial folds, is a known hallmark of lupus; although it may be confused with rosacea or polymorphous light eruption. The malar rash with autoantibodies, particularly ANA (almost 100% sensitive), and anti-double stranded DNA (95% specific), will lend themselves to a conclusive diagnosis [22]. Nonetheless, it should be noted that research criteria is not necessary for a diagnosis of lupus. The research criterion is merely a tool, used to randomize patients into homogeneous groups, while in fact physicians are treating a heterogeneous disease. So, in the quest to stratify patients by nonskilled physicians, or those not comfortable diagnosing or treating lupus properly, diagnostic criteria is often helpful, but certainly cannot be the quintessential element of a lupus diagnosis. In reality, actually "labeling" a patient with a lupus diagnosis may require a protracted course. Theoretically, a patient may carry a label of unspecified connective tissue disease (UCTD) for some time, before a conclusive diagnosis can be given. In time, this patient may develop lupus, Sjogren's syndrome, rheumatoid arthritis, scleroderma, myositis, an overlap syndrome, anti-synthetase syndrome, Sjogren's syndrome, IgG4-related disease, or sarcoid.

2.2 Consider evidence of lupus in every disease

Physicians should consider lupus as every disease they see, and work backward from that point. Note the following:

1. When a patient presents with hair loss (i.e., a bald spot - non-scarring alopecia); the differential diagnoses are broad and lupus should be investigated, the patient will need to be followed and skin biopsies performed [23].

2. Lesions, such as discoid lupus, which are characteristic scaly lesions, discolored, typically hyper-pigmented, and located within the ears, are common

Positive antinuclear antibody (ANA)	97%
Malaise and fatigue	90%
Arthralgia, myalgia	90%
Sun sensitivity, skin changes	70%
Cognitive dysfunction	70%
Low C3 or C4 complement	61%
Fever due to lupus	57%
Antibodies to ds DNA	50%
Arthritis	50%
Leukopenia	46%
Pleuritis	44%
Anemia	42%
Alopecia	40%
Nephritis, proteinuria	40%
Anticardiolipin antibody	35%
Malar rash	35%
Central nervous system	32%
Increased gamma globulin	32%
Weight loss due to lupus	27%
Raynaud's	25%
Hypertension	25%
Sjogren's	25%
Oral ulcerations (mouth, nose)	20%
Discoid lesions	20%
Central nervous system vasculitis	15%
Adenopathy	15%
Pleural effusion	12%
Subacute cutaneous lupus	10%
Myositis	10%
Avascular necrosis	10%

Table 1.
Approximate prevalence (%) of selected symptoms, signs, and laboratory abnormalities of systemic lupus erythematosus during the course of the disease in the United States [29].

in lupus [24]. Although these lesions may be seen in other conditions, lupus should be considered.

3. Uveitis, typically anterior, is common in lupus [25]. It may occur one time, and may be infectious. Diagnostic possibilities included syphilis, tuberculosis or Lyme disease. If these infections are excluded, then undoubtedly, even if the patient's uveitis is a first-time occurrence, a lupus workup should be initiated.

As with all patients presenting any of the above features, clinicians should initiate confirmatory laboratory workup, including phospholipids, ANA, DNA, ENA, SSA, and SSB, in order to establish a baseline, when a patient exhibits a potential lupus feature at any point. Hypothetically a young patient, between 15 and 20 years of age, may present to a clinic with anterior uveitis. Rather than labeling this as viral, the practitioner should immediately consider a differential diagnosis that includes lupus. Other differential possibilities would include syphilis, tuberculosis, HLA-B27 diseases (including but not limited to psoriatic arthritis), HLA-B27 uveitis, ankylosing spondylitis, reactive arthritis, Crohn's colitis and ulcerative colitis. Regardless of the ultimate diagnosis, the treatment does not change; however, if the patient requires treatment with hydroxychloroquine, early diagnosis may lead to a more favorable outcome. Hydroxychloroquine is paramount. Many clinical trials over decades support its efficacy in prevention of lupus flares, thrombosis in lupus patients, and lipid-lowering potential [26].

In addition to the three presentations listed above, mouth sores also occur in lupus, Crohn's disease, Behcet's disease, phospholipid antibody syndrome, tuberculosis, syphilis, sarcoidosis, Sjogren's syndrome, IgG4-related disease, and viral infections [27]. Viral ulcers tend to be painful. Behcet's ulcers generally reveal large, circumscribed, beefy-red borders. Ulcers associated with Crohn's disease are usually shallow painful ulcers, similar to those seen in sarcoidosis. Lupus ulcers are frequently painless and often noticed surreptitiously [28].

Additionally, isolated lymphadenopathy does not necessarily have to be hilar or mediastinal; it could be epitrochlear, glandular swelling, lacrimal, parotid, or submandibular. However, the finding, incidental or not, with or without dry eyes and dry mouth, may be an indication of lupus (**Table 1**).

3. Common presentations of lupus

The following represents selected symptoms and abnormalities in patients diagnosed with lupus within in the United States.

3.1 Arthropathies

Approximately 50% of lupus patients suffer from arthritis [29]. Joint disease, quite often a small joint polyarthritis, typically symmetric, is noted with typical involvement of PIPs, MCPs and wrists, inflammatory in nature; however, this is not erosive, which differentiates it from rheumatoid arthritis [30]. However, the practitioner should keep in mind that the differential diagnosis of IgG4-related disease, lymphomas, Sjogren's, sarcoidosis, or spondyloarthropathies, can also present with a phenotypic appearance of lupus arthritis. The definitive finding of arthritis only seen in lupus would be lupus arthropathy or acute rheumatic fever, which is followed by Jaccoud's arthropathy. Jaccoud's arthropathy is a chronic, non-erosive, reversible (with proper splinting) joint disorder that may occur after repeated bouts of arthritis. This arthropathy is caused by inflammation of the joint capsule and subsequent fibrotic retraction, causing ulnar deviation of the fingers, through metacarpophalangeal joint subluxation, primarily of the fourth and fifth fingers [31].

The greatest emphasis should be placed on the fact that all joints could be involved in lupus. Arthritis of lupus may be the presenting feature, and therefore, all cases of inflammatory arthritis must be evaluated with x-rays and a thorough history and physical, to exclude other diseases. Treatment would begin with the use of hydroxychloroquine and the addition of methotrexate. If necessary, abatacept (a CTLA4 inhibitor drug), could be added, as well as the newer medication discussed earlier, belimumab. Additionally, low dose steroids are often effective. While some practitioners may view steroids as poison, others feel the patient's quality of life, on Prednisone (5 mg or less), even permanently could be appropriate, if this is necessary for disease control and improvement in the patient's quality of life. The patient should be informed of necessity for vigilance with regard to sleep, lipid and blood pressure monitoring, and the risk of osteoporosis. In the final analysis, the ratio of logic needs to be brought into consideration. As a practicing rheumatologist, with a personal experience of 32 years, experience dictates that 5 mg of Prednisone or less in virtually all the inflammatory patients that cannot be weaned, failed to cause significant steroid side effects. In the minority of patients who do suffer steroid side effects from a 5 mg daily equivalent or less as they begin to age, skin fragility or perhaps early cataracts can be seen; however, this may be difficult to ascertain, unless their ophthalmologist is convinced that any posterior subscapular cataract is the definite consequence of steroid use. Otherwise, this would be difficult to ascertain [32].

3.2 Thrombocytopenia/thrombocytosis

Approximately 42–46% of patients develop a cytopenia, including leukopenia and anemia [29]. Cytopenias in lupus are typically recognized with anemia, often hemolytic or of chronic disease, thrombocytopenia, or thrombocytosis [33]. Thrombocytosis indicates inflammation, while thrombocytopenia is often autoimmune and antiplatelet antibodies lower platelet counts; however, this should not be taken for granted. As in Sjogren's, the mechanism would be hypersplenism; however, the finding of thrombocytopenia must prompt a probe for lupus. This protocol also stands in the case of a low white blood cell count. A WBC less than 4000 units for all, or lymphocyte of less than 1000, should both prompt an evaluation and workup for lupus. These findings while not specific are quite typical. Please note that one isolated sample needs repeating.

3.3 Lupus nephritis

Approximately 40% of lupus patients are diagnosed with nephritis [29]. The patient presents with blood or protein in the urine [34]. A renal biopsy is performed. A diagnosis is established - Mesangial proliferative, diffuse or focal proliferation, or pure membranous. The treatments for this vary. The current main stay treatment is mycophenolate mofetil. A new medication, which will be available in the near future, is calcineurin inhibitor, Voclasporin [35]. The data regarding this is promising. Rituximab, anecdotally, and in Pureview Data, indicates that it may also be helpful, although it is not the standard of care. Emphasis should be placed on the actuality that "the standard of care" should supersede the Food and Drug Administration's indications for any drug. Approval for a drug by the Food and Drug Administration is solely based on the drug company's actual "indication application" for that particular drug. While it may be used exclusively for its indication, in some cases it should be noted that the drug may prove more effective for off label use. This unfortunately seems to be a matter of "dollars and cents" where the pharmaceutical companies are concerned when determining the indication, they seek from the FDA.

3.4 Central nervous system

Roughly 32% of lupus patients develop lupus that attacks the central nervous system [29]. Lupus involving the central nervous system is both a confusing and interesting aspect of the disease [36, 37]. Virtually any central nervous system or peripheral nervous system problem including, but not limited to, neuropathy, mononeuritis multiplex, seizures, blindness, loss of hearing, cranial nerve palsy, encephalopathy, psychosis and movement disorders, are not uncommon in the lupus population, and may frequently present as an initial feature of the disease.

To reemphasize, all symptomatology that has been mentioned in this chapter may be an initial feature of lupus; however, the lack of swift rheumatology involvement often ultimately leads to a delay in diagnosis, which is always detrimental to the patient. Therefore, it is important to perform a comprehensive evaluation, including biopsy, angiogram, or other internal organ imaging, as well as complete serologic testing. Additionally, most patients are not willing to take medication for extended periods of time, unless it can be proven to them by their physician that the medication will indeed benefit them by alleviating the symptoms they are experiencing. This will assist in a more accurate diagnosis of lupus versus another disease process. As in every case involving a possible autoimmune process, emphasis should be placed on the importance of swift initiation of workup, as this will facilitate the timely establishment of proper treatment.

If a patient is acutely ill with psychosis, they will typically be treated in a hospital setting, being initially seen by neurology and psychiatry, as other specialists. Unfortunately, this occurs before a rheumatologist is consulted [38]. An immediate MRI of the brain and lumbar puncture should be ordered, along with autoantibodies and cerebrospinal fluid, to assess the ribosomal P antibody, GAD65 antibody and NMO. With these proper evaluations, the likelihood of a CNS lupus diagnosis may be determined.

It is quite typical in that lupus patients, including those with renal and central nervous system involvement, in general, do quite well with medical compliance. Published death rates, transplant rates, and dialysis rates for lupus nephritis are decidedly dependent upon the population type that is investigated. A well-educated compliant group of patients has a very low incidence of end stage renal disease while the noncompliant group almost certainly ultimately develop end stage renal disease [39].

3.5 Abdominal pain

Another presentation would be abdominal pain, rather than splenomegaly. This would account for approximately 27% of lupus symptomatology [29]. A patient with severe abdominal pain, who is known to have lupus, after a proper workup for exclusion of perforated viscus or ischemic disease, the treatment would be steroids for what is mesenteric arteritis or serositis. The prognosis would not change, as they are both treated with moderate high dose steroids, oral or IV. Again, this can be a presenting feature of lupus. To the detriment of the patient, they are often are seen by gastroenterologists, who run a plethora of tests, including CTAs and MRIs of various organs, only to ultimately discover a case of hepatosplenomegaly with pain. At that point, to the misfortune of the patient, unnecessary surgery is generally performed for the hepatosplenomegaly, and sadly, the patient passes away as a result. If the patient had been treated properly, their life could have been saved, as they would have been successfully treated with 1 to 2 mg/kg of prednisolone or similar [40].

3.6 Pancreatitis and Raynaud's phenomenon

Pancreatitis is an excellent example of a disease, which is not part of the listed diagnostic criteria for lupus. Raynaud's phenomenon also not listed in the diagnostic criteria, although approximately 25% of lupus patients suffer from this condition [29, 41]. While either of those may be the presenting feature of systemic lupus, neither are listed as diagnostic criteria which is fine; however, the practitioner should perform a thorough workup to determine if a patient who has pancreatitis, as they may well have lupus. It should be noted however, that alcoholism, gallstone disease and pancreatic divisum, without the atypical sausage pancreas of IgG4-related disease, must be ruled out.

With regard to Raynaud's, the reversible spasm of vessels, usually induced by cold or emotional provocation, typically with triple phase color response from 5 to 60 minutes, is a frequent feature in lupus patients and may well be the initial finding of the disease. The practitioner must look past scleroderma, which has a more ominous prognosis than Raynaud's related to lupus. This is often differentiated with a simple in-office nailfold capillaroscopy, which by in large, is a tremendously underutilized tool [42]. For the well-seasoned rheumatologist, this technique is used more often, but it should be used with regularity. In fact, nailfold capillaroscopy should be used as a baseline in all potential cases of autoimmune patients.

3.7 Heart and lungs

Attention to the heart and lungs is essential [43]. A patient with recurrent pneumonias is more likely to have lupus pneumonitis or an autoinflammatory disease, rather than the occurrence of infectious pneumonia every three months. After the onset of a second case of pneumonia, a rheumatologist should be consulted, but commonly, this does not occur. Regrettably, the patient who is suffering from an autoimmune disease has now suffered without a proper diagnosis for an unspecified amount of time. At this point, it would be advantageous to the patient to be seen by a rheumatologist without further delay.

Other common heart and lung manifestations of lupus include pleurisy and/or pericardial effusion [44]. Approximately 12% of lupus patients will develop a pericardial effusion [29]. Alarmingly, in several medical institutions, the treatment of choice for pericardial effusion is a pericardial window. Unfortunately, as in the case of inappropriate splenectomy with abdominal pain in a case of lupus, as mentioned earlier, a pericardial window is carries equal efficacy in a lupus patient presenting with pericardial effusion. As there is no indication for abdominal surgery for a patient with lupus abdominal pain, there is also virtually no indication for pericardial window in a lupus pericarditis patient. The incidence of tamponade is extraordinarily low. Myxomatosis valvular heart disease or so-called Libman-Sacks endocarditis, with or without phospholipid antibodies, is another finding that should be noted, although this is often woefully overlooked.

3.8 Overlooked autoimmunity

Many lupus patients suffer from autoimmunity that is frequently overlooked and therefore; the percentage of sufferers remains uncalculated [45]. The most common is likely Hashimoto's thyroid disease; however, other conditions include Graves' disease, myasthenia gravis, Addison's disease, primary biliary cirrhosis, and autoimmune hepatitis. Each of these has autoimmune associations that should not be overlooked. Many of the features potentially seen in Sjogren's syndrome, or many lupus-like features such as interstitial lung disease, should never be taken for granted based on the positive ANA or research criteria, as those patients may well have myositis or scleroderma. As mentioned in Part 2 of this chapter, "A Rheum with a Different View", lupus should be considered in every disease.

4. The thought process of a rheumatologist

There are deep gaps between the thought process and treatment plans of a rheumatologist versus that of a general internist, family practitioner, ophthalmologist, or orthopedic surgeon or any other practitioner involved in a patient's care.

Rheumatology remains greatly underutilized. This regrettably adds substantial delay to the diagnosis and treatment of a patient. It bears mentioning again that all organ systems may be involved in lupus. Based on this, the all-purpose criteria is preferable to the new SLICC criteria for diagnosis of lupus, as it was far more practical [46]. It also bears mentioning again that no practitioner may diagnose lupus, or any other disease process, based solely on research criteria. Criteria are to be used merely as a guideline. For example, a patient presents to their physician, stating they are "not feeling well". Subsequently, blood studies are ordered that reveal an ANA with a very high titer and upon further perusal, a very high DNA is also discovered, yet the physician fails to recognize that this patient has a forme-fruste of lupus. A rheumatologist would have started the patient on Plaquenil and educated them with regard to their diagnosis, and the physical ramifications to expect in the future.

Two of the most interesting, but also difficult to treat diseases, a physician may encounter include pulmonary renal syndrome, presenting with alveolar hemorrhage, and glomerular nephritis with ANA, DNA, successfully treated with cyclophosphamide [47]. Another rare, but not uncommon complication of lupus, would be TTP with or without the ADAMTS13 gene and ocular inflammation and orbital pseudotumor. Consider the case of a patient who presented with true renal failure, visual hallucinations and movement disorder. At that point the patient was treated with IV Cytoxan and pulse steroids. Therefore, the patient did not have fever; however the patient was anemic and had schistocytes with an elevated reticulocyte count. Thus, the patient did not fulfill all of the criteria for TTP; therefore, a clinical diagnosis was made of the same. The patient responded almost immediately to with all features of the disease disappearing with plasma exchange. This is a wonderful case to recall, when a hematologist says to a patient, "It cannot be TTP because there is no fever", apparently, this hematologist has lost sight of the fact that the high dose steroids likely blunted the fever. They may argue that there are not enough schistocytes [48] to fulfill the bacteria, however when schistocytes should not exist, and anemia cannot be explained, it can only be rationalized that the use of cyclophosphamides and high dose steroids lowered the schistocytes [49, 50]. This is a fantastic example of why research criteria alone, should never be used for diagnostic purposes.

It is very important to understand the mechanism of action for each disease feature, as it will impact a patient's treatment. For the purpose of example, thrombocytopenia will be seen in Sjogren's syndrome and hypersplenism, while in lupus platelet antibodies, both conditions can be present with dry eyes and dry mouth. A salivary gland biopsy may not differentiate, as a positive lymphocyte score of 50 lymphocytes $4mm^2$, may presumably be seen in either condition. This may lead to an overlap diagnosis, or based on the mechanism of thrombocytopenia, it may also sway the diagnosis. Pneumonitis, while common in lupus, is seen in other autoimmune diseases, including sarcoidosis. All conditions mentioned may have a positive rheumatoid factor or positive ANA. Even CCP antibodies can be seen in autoimmune diseases with low values [51].

5. Conclusions

Lupus is a great mimicker. This is due in part to a woeful lack of knowledge by most practitioners, as well as the absence of specific treatments. However, based on our available knowledge, with earlier institution of proper rheumatologic assistance, patients would be diagnosed with greater accuracy and proper treatments begun in a timely manner. Also, with patient compliance, education and understanding outcome is better reference. Consulting a rheumatologist promptly, would not only benefit the patient, but also profit the medical system by eradicating useless tests and treatment options that are often unmerited. Unfortunately, in a world of protocol, many are afraid to take an unconventional approach. It is because of this; other physicians often fail to consider a rheumatologic consultation [52].

Author details

Stephen Soloway[1,2]

1 Arthritis and Rheumatology Associates of South Jersey, P.C., Vineland, NJ, USA

2 Chief of Rheumatology, Inspira Medical Network, Mullica Hill and Vineland, NJ, USA

*Address all correspondence to: cdipaola@drsoloway.com

References

[1] Kuhn A, Bonsmann G, Anders HJ, Herzer P, Tenbrock K, Schneider M. The Diagnosis and Treatment of Systemic Lupus Erythematosus. Dtsch Arztebl Int. 2015 Jun 19;112(25):423-32. doi: 10.3238/arztebl.2015.0423. PMID: 26179016; PMCID: PMC4558874.

[2] Wallace, Daniel J. (Daniel Jeffrey), 1949-The lupus book : a guide for patients and their families / Daniel J. Wallace. – 5th ed.

[3] Tunnicliffe DJ, Palmer SC, Henderson L, Masson P, Craig JC, Tong A, Singh-Grewal D, Flanc RS, Roberts MA, Webster AC, Strippoli GF. Immunosuppressive treatment for proliferative lupus nephritis. Cochrane Database Syst Rev. 2018 Jun 29;6(6):CD002922. doi: 10.1002/14651858.CD002922.pub4. PMID: 29957821; PMCID: PMC6513226.

[4] Felten R, Scher F, Sagez F, Chasset F, Arnaud L. Spotlight on anifrolumab and its potential for the treatment of moderate-to-severe systemic lupus erythematosus: evidence to date. Drug Des Devel Ther. 2019 May 8;13:1535-1543. doi: 10.2147/DDDT.S170969. PMID: 31190735; PMCID: PMC6514126.

[5] Baigrie D, Bansal P, Goyal A, Crane JS. Leukocytoclastic Vasculitis. 2020 Aug 11. In: StatPearls [Internet]. Treasure Island (FL): StatPearls Publishing; 2020 Jan–. PMID: 29489227.

[6] Qiao W, Ding H, Zuo Y, Jiang L, Zhou J, Han X, Yu L, Du R, M Hedrich C, Deng GM. Lupus IgG deposition causes arthritis but inhibits bone destruction through competitive occupation of FcγRI and reduced RANKL signalling. Clin Transl Immunology. 2020 Sep 6;9(9):e1174. doi: 10.1002/cti2.1174. PMID: 32994999; PMCID: PMC7507387.

[7] Komolafe OO. Rapidly progressive glomerulonephritis: A wild card manifestation of lupus nephritis. Saudi J Kidney Dis Transpl. 2018 Mar-Apr;29(2):443-451. doi: 10.4103/1319-2442.229293. PMID: 29657218.

[8] Rutgers A, Sanders JS, Stegeman CA, Kallenberg CG. Pauci-immune necrotizing glomerulonephritis. Rheum Dis Clin North Am. 2010 Aug;36(3):559-572. doi: 10.1016/j.rdc.2010.05.002. PMID: 20688250.

[9] DeVrieze BW, Hurley JA. Goodpasture Syndrome. 2020 Mar 25. In: StatPearls [Internet]. Treasure Island (FL): StatPearls Publishing; 2020 Jan–. PMID: 29083697.

[10] Mustaqeem R, Arif A. Renal Tubular Acidosis. 2020 Aug 16. In: StatPearls [Internet]. Treasure Island (FL): StatPearls Publishing; 2020 Jan–. PMID: 30085586.

[11] Muriithi AK, Leung N, Valeri AM, et al. Biopsy-proven acute interstitial nephritis, 1993-2011: a case series. Am J Kidney Dis 2014;64:558-566.

[12] Cortazar FB, Kibbelaar ZA, Glezerman IG, et al. Clinical features and outcomes of immune checkpoint inhibitor-associated AKI: a multicenter study. J Am Soc Nephrol 2020;31: 435-446.

[13] Huong DL, Papo T, Beaufils H, et al. Renal involvement in systemic lupus erythematosus: a study of 180 patients from a single center. Medicine (Baltimore) 1999;78:148-166.

[14] Yu F, Wu L-H, Tan Y, et al. Tubulo-interstitial lesions of patients with lupus nephritis classified by the 2003 International Society of Nephrology and Renal Pathology Society system. Kidney Int 2010;77:820-829.

[15] Cortazar FB, Stone JH. IgG4-related disease and the kidney. Nat Rev Nephrol 2015;11:599-609.

[16] Raissian Y, Nasr SH, Larsen CP, et al. Diagnosis of IgG4-related tubulointerstitial nephritis. J Am Soc Nephrol 2011;22:1343-1352.

[17] McCabe C, Jones Q, Nikolopoulou A, Wathen C, Luqmani R. Pulmonary-renal syndromes: an update for respiratory physicians. Respir Med. 2011 Oct;105(10):1413-1421. doi: 10.1016/j.rmed.2011.05.012. PMID: 21684732.

[18] Jennette JC, Nachman PH. ANCA Glomerulonephritis and Vasculitis. Clin J Am Soc Nephrol. 2017 Oct 6;12(10):1680-1691. doi: 10.2215/CJN.02500317. Epub 2017 Aug 25. PMID: 28842398; PMCID: PMC5628710.

[19] Saccucci M, Di Carlo G, Bossù M, Giovarruscio F, Salucci A, Polimeni A. Autoimmune Diseases and Their Manifestations on Oral Cavity: Diagnosis and Clinical Management. J Immunol Res. 2018 May 27;2018:6061825. doi: 10.1155/2018/6061825. PMID: 29977929; PMCID: PMC5994274.

[20] Andrews JS, Trupin L, Schmajuk G, Barton J, Margaretten M, Yazdany J, Yelin EH, Katz PP. Muscle Strength and Changes in Physical Function in Women With Systemic Lupus Erythematosus. Arthritis Care Res (Hoboken). 2015 Aug;67(8):1070-7. doi: 10.1002/acr.22560. PMID: 25623919; PMCID: PMC4515406.

[21] Lee KC, Ladizinski B, Federman DG. Complications associated with use of levamisole-contaminated cocaine: an emerging public health challenge. Mayo Clin Proc. 2012 Jun;87(6):581-6. doi: 10.1016/j.mayocp.2012.03.010. PMID: 22677078; PMCID: PMC3498128.

[22] Vasquez-Canizares N, Wahezi D, Putterman C. Diagnostic and prognostic tests in systemic lupus erythematosus. Best Pract Res Clin Rheumatol. 2017 Jun;31(3):351-363. doi: 10.1016/j.berh.2017.10.002. Epub 2017 Nov 6. PMID: 29224677; PMCID: PMC5776716.

[23] Chanprapaph K, Udompanich S, Visessiri Y, Ngamjanyaporn P, Suchonwanit P. Nonscarring alopecia in systemic lupus erythematosus: A cross-sectional study with trichoscopic, histopathologic, and immunopathologic analyses. J Am Acad Dermatol. 2019 Dec;81(6):1319-1329. doi: 10.1016/j.jaad.2019.05.053. Epub 2019 May 28. PMID: 31150712.

[24] Jefferson GD, Aakalu VK, Braniecki M. Tumid lupus: An unexpected diagnosis for the otolaryngologist. Am J Otolaryngol. 2017 Mar-Apr;38(2):257-259. doi: 10.1016/j.amjoto.2017.01.003. Epub 2017 Jan 17. PMID: 28122678; PMCID: PMC5826658.

[25] Klímová A, Seidler Štangová P, Svozílková P, Kučera T, Heissigerová J. Klinicképrojevyexperimentálníautoimunitní uveitidy [The Clinical Signs of Experimental Autoimmune Uveitis]. Cesk Slov Oftalmol. 2016 Feb;72(1):276-82. Czech. PMID: 27041283.

[26] Tao CY, Shang J, Chen T, Yu D, Jiang YM, Liu D, Cheng GY, Xiao J, Zhao ZZ. Impact of antimalarial (AM) on serum lipids in systemic lupus erythematosus (SLE) patients: A systematic review and meta-analysis. Medicine (Baltimore). 2019 Apr;98(14):e15030. doi: 10.1097/MD.0000000000015030. PMID: 30946340; PMCID: PMC6456110.

[27] Chi AC, Neville BW, Krayer JW, Gonsalves WC. Oral manifestations of systemic disease. Am Fam Physician. 2010 Dec 1;82(11):1381-1388. PMID: 21121523.

[28] Carubbi F, Alunno A, Gerli R, Giacomelli R. Histopathology of salivary glands. Reumatismo. 2018 Oct 3;70(3):146-154. doi: 10.4081/reumatismo.2018.1053. PMID: 30282440.\

[29] Wallace, Daniel J. (Daniel Jeffrey), 1949-The lupus book : a guide for patients and their families / Daniel J. Wallace. – 5th ed.

[30] Ceccarelli F, Perricone C, Cipriano E, Massaro L, Natalucci F, Capalbo G, Leccese I, Bogdanos D, Spinelli FR, Alessandri C, Valesini G, Conti F. Joint involvement in systemic lupus erythematosus: From pathogenesis to clinical assessment. Semin Arthritis Rheum. 2017 Aug;47(1):53-64. doi: 10.1016/j.semarthrit.2017.03.022. Epub 2017 Apr 4. PMID: 28465078.

[31] van Vugt RM, Derksen RH, Kater L, Bijlsma JW. Deforming arthropathy or lupus and rhupus hands in systemic lupus erythematosus. Ann Rheum Dis. 1998 Sep;57(9):540-4. doi: 10.1136/ard.57.9.540. PMID: 9849313; PMCID: PMC1752746.

[32] Kabadi S, Yeaw J, Bacani AK, Tafesse E, Bos K, Karkare S, DeKoven M, Vina ER. Healthcare resource utilization and costs associated with long-term corticosteroid exposure in patients with systemic lupus erythematosus. Lupus. 2018 Oct;27(11):1799-1809. doi: 10.1177/0961203318790675. Epub 2018 Aug 1. PMID: 30068254; PMCID: PMC6264911.

[33] Brierley CK, Pavord S. Autoimmune cytopenias and thrombotic thrombocytopenic purpura. Clin Med (Lond). 2018 Aug;18(4):335-339. doi: 10.7861/clinmedicine.18-4-335. PMID: 30072561; PMCID: PMC6334040.

[34] Chimenti MS, Di Stefani A, Conigliaro P, Saggini A, Urbani S, Giunta A, Esposito M, Bianchi L, Peris K, Perricone R. Histopathology of the skin in rheumatic diseases. Reumatismo. 2018 Oct 3;70(3):187-198. doi: 10.4081/reumatismo.2018.1049. PMID: 30282444.

[35] Jessop S, Whitelaw DA, Grainge MJ, Jayasekera P. Drugs for discoid lupus erythematosus. Cochrane Database Syst Rev. 2017 May 5;5(5):CD002954. doi: 10.1002/14651858.CD002954.pub3. PMID: 28476075; PMCID: PMC6481466.

[36] Hanly JG, Kozora E, Beyea SD, Birnbaum J. Review: Nervous System Disease in Systemic Lupus Erythematosus: Current Status and Future Directions. Arthritis Rheumatol. 2019 Jan;71(1):33-42. doi: 10.1002/art.40591. Epub 2018 Nov 24. PMID: 29927108.

[37] Kivity S, Agmon-Levin N, Zandman-Goddard G, Chapman J, Shoenfeld Y. Neuropsychiatric lupus: a mosaic of clinical presentations. BMC Med. 2015 Mar 4;13:43. doi: 10.1186/s12916-015-0269-8. PMID: 25858312; PMCID: PMC4349748.

[38] Hanly JG, Li Q, Su L, Urowitz MB, Gordon C, Bae SC, Romero-Diaz J, Sanchez-Guerrero J, Bernatsky S, Clarke AE, Wallace DJ, Isenberg DA, Rahman A, Merrill JT, Fortin PR, Gladman DD, Bruce IN, Petri M, Ginzler EM, Dooley MA, Steinsson K, Ramsey-Goldman R, Zoma AA, Manzi S, Nived O, Jonsen A, Khamashta MA, Alarcón GS, van Vollenhoven RF, Aranow C, Mackay M, Ruiz-Irastorza G, Ramos-Casals M, Lim SS, Inanc M, Kalunian KC, Jacobsen S, Peschken CA, Kamen DL, Askanase A, Theriault C, Farewell V. Psychosis in Systemic Lupus Erythematosus: Results From an International Inception Cohort Study. Arthritis Rheumatol. 2019 Feb;71(2):281-289. doi: 10.1002/art.40764. Epub 2019 Jan 18. PMID: 30375754; PMCID: PMC6353684.

[39] Tesar V, Hruskova Z. Lupus Nephritis: A Different Disease in European Patients? Kidney Dis (Basel). 2015 Sep;1(2):110-8. doi: 10.1159/000438844. Epub 2015 Aug 28. PMID: 27536671; PMCID: PMC4934820.

[40] Adler BL, Timlin H, Birnbaum J. Lupus intestinal pseudo-obstruction and hydronephrosis: Case report. Medicine (Baltimore). 2019 Jul;98(28):e16178. doi: 10.1097/MD.0000000000016178. PMID: 31305400; PMCID: PMC6641825.

[41] Hesselstrand R, Iagnocco A, Kayser C, Melsens K, Müller-Ladner U,

Paolino S, Pizzorni C, Radic M, Riccieri V, Snow M, Stevens W, Sulli A, van Laar JM, Vonk MC, Vanhaecke A, Cutolo M; EULAR Study Group on Microcirculation in Rheumatic Diseases and the Scleroderma Clinical Trials Consortium Group on Capillaroscopy. Standardisation of nailfold capillaroscopy for the assessment of patients with Raynaud's phenomenon and systemic sclerosis. Autoimmun Rev. 2020 Mar;19(3):102458. doi: 10.1016/j.autrev.2020.102458. Epub 2020 Jan 10. PMID: 31927087.

[42] Smith V, Herrick AL, Ingegnoli F, Damjanov N, De Angelis R, Denton CP, Distler O, Espejo K, Foeldvari I, Frech T, Garro B, Gutierrez M, Gyger G, Hachulla E, Hesselstrand R, Iagnocco A, Kayser C, Melsens K, Müller-Ladner U, Paolino S, Pizzorni C, Radic M, Riccieri V, Snow M, Stevens W, Sulli A, van Laar JM, Vonk MC, Vanhaecke A, Cutolo M; EULAR Study Group on Microcirculation in Rheumatic Diseases and the Scleroderma Clinical Trials Consortium Group on Capillaroscopy. Standardisation of nailfold capillaroscopy for the assessment of patients with Raynaud's phenomenon and systemic sclerosis. Autoimmun Rev. 2020 Mar;19(3):102458. doi: 10.1016/j.autrev.2020.102458. Epub 2020 Jan 10. PMID: 31927087.

[43] Signorini V, Elefante E, Zucchi D, Trentin F, Bortoluzzi A, Tani C. One year in review 2020: systemic lupus erythematosus. Clin Exp Rheumatol. 2020 Jul-Aug;38(4):592-601. Epub 2020 Jul 10. PMID: 32662410.

[44] Bezwada P, Quadri A, Shaikh A, Ayala-Rodriguez C, Green S. Myopericarditis and Pericardial Effusion as the Initial Presentation of Systemic Lupus Erythematosus. Case Rep Med. 2017;2017:6912020. doi: 10.1155/2017/6912020. Epub 2017 Feb 5. PMID: 28261271; PMCID: PMC5316435.

[45] Basta F, Fasola F, Triantafyllias K, Schwarting A. Systemic Lupus Erythematosus (SLE) Therapy: The Old and the New. Rheumatol Ther. 2020 Sep;7(3):433-446. doi: 10.1007/s40744-020-00212-9. Epub 2020 Jun 2. PMID: 32488652; PMCID: PMC7410873.

[46] Tiao J, Feng R, Carr K, Okawa J, Werth VP. Using the American College of Rheumatology (ACR) and Systemic Lupus International Collaborating Clinics (SLICC) criteria to determine the diagnosis of systemic lupus erythematosus (SLE) in patients with subacute cutaneous lupus erythematosus (SCLE). J Am Acad Dermatol. 2016 May;74(5):862-9. doi: 10.1016/j.jaad.2015.12.029. Epub 2016 Feb 18. PMID: 26897388; PMCID: PMC4879000.

[47] Nasser M, Cottin V. The Respiratory System in Autoimmune Vascular Diseases. Respiration. 2018;96(1):12-28. doi: 10.1159/000486899. Epub 2018 Jul 4. PMID: 29975964.

[48] Nasser M, Cottin V. The Respiratory System in Autoimmune Vascular Diseases. Respiration. 2018;96(1):12-28. doi: 10.1159/000486899. Epub 2018 Jul 4. PMID: 29975964.

[49] Schapkaitz E, Mezgebe MH. The Clinical Significance of Schistocytes: A Prospective Evaluation of the International Council for Standardization in Hematology Schistocyte Guidelines. Turk J Haematol. 2017 Mar 1;34(1):59-63. doi: 10.4274/tjh.2016.0359. Epub 2016 Oct 31. PMID: 27795225; PMCID: PMC5451690.

[50] Chiasakul T, Cuker A. Clinical and laboratory diagnosis of TTP: an integrated approach. Hematology Am Soc Hematol Educ Program. 2018 Nov 30;2018(1):530-538. doi: 10.1182/asheducation-2018.1.530. PMID: 30504354; PMCID: PMC6246034.

[51] Soloway A, Late-onset Systemic Lupus Erythematosus Presenting with Pneumonitis and Class IV Lupus

Nephritis, 2019 ACP Poster Contest Winner NYS

[52] Hoover PJ, Costenbader KH. Insights into the epidemiology and management of lupus nephritis from the US rheumatologist's perspective. Kidney Int. 2016 Sep;90(3):487-92. doi: 10.1016/j.kint.2016.03.042. Epub 2016 Jun 22. PMID: 27344205; PMCID: PMC5679458.

Section 2

The Lupus Kidney Disease Update

Chapter 2

Lupus Nephritis: Renal Biopsy Guiding the Clinician

Rosa Marlene Viero and Daniela Cristina dos Santos

Abstract

Systemic lupus erythematosus is a chronic autoimmune disease that affects mostly women. The kidneys are involved in 50% of patients causing a high degree of disease morbidity and mortality with poor prognosis. Early diagnosis of lupus nephritis with prompt therapy correlates with a better outcome. The renal biopsy provides important informations to clinicians to monitor the patients. The patterns of glomerular lesion, degree of activity and chronicity of the disease and extent of lesions to the tubulointerstitial and vascular compartments are fundamental information for the clinician to decide the most appropriate treatment. In order to correlate the kidney disease with clinical manifestations and patient outcome the glomerular lesions are classified according to International Society of Nephrology and Renal Pathology Society Classification (ISN/RPS). The definition of active and chronic lesions was introduced by studies conducted at National Institute of Health (NIH). The ISN/RPS classification and NIH indices have recently been revised by a series of retrospective validation studies to improve and minimize the controversial aspects.

Keywords: Systemic lupus erithematosus, lupus nephritis, renal biopsy, ISN/RPS classification, NIH activity and chronicity indices, patients management, prognosis

1. Introduction

Systemic lupus erythematosus (SLE) is a chronic multisystem autoimmune disease that frequently involve kidneys in women. The development of the disease is related to exposure to environmental factors in individuals with genetic predisposition. It is characterized by loss of tolerance against nuclear autoantigens, lymphoproliferation, polyclonal autoantibody production, immune complex disease and multiorgan tissue inflammation [1]. The affected organs include skin, joints, heart, lungs, kidneys, central nervous system and serous membranes. The disease involves a sequence of manifestations such as arthritis, serositis, chronic fatigue, skin rashes, glomerulonephritis, neurological involvement and hematological abnormalities [2]. SLE is the most frequent cause of secondary glomerular disease [3–5]. Lupus nephritis (LN) as a disease usually develops early in the clinical course of SLE in up to 50% of patients. The development of effective diagnostic tests and the introduction of new therapies has shown an improvement in the survival of patients with SLE. However, SLE patients still have a higher risk of death than the general population, especially patients with LN. Lupus glomerulonephritis with intense activity requires greater immunosuppression with increased risk of death from opportunistic infections. On the other hand, long-term treatment with high-dose of corticosteroids is a risk factor for coronary atherosclerosis and cardiovascular disease [1, 6]. Glomerular immune complexes can activate complement and engage leukocyte Fc receptors to initiate renal inflammation and injury [1]. LN has very pleomorphic clinical and morphologic expressions. Clinical findings range from asymptomatic hematuria and proteinuria to nephrotic syndrome or rapidly progressive renal failure [7].

2. Renal biopsy

The renal biopsy is the gold standard for the diagnosis of LN, providing important information to the clinician for the management of the patients [7–9]. A diagnosis of SLE is based on clinical systemic features and serologic tests attending the American College of Rheumatology (ACR) criteria for SLE [10]. However, it is not uncommon that the renal biopsy shows morphologic expressions that is very suspicious or conclusive of LN before extrarenal manifestations are evident [11]. The renal biopsy provides an important information about the morphology and severity of the lesions, their classification, grades of activity and chronicity of the disease. With the appearance of any signs or symptoms of kidney disease such as hematuria, proteinuria, nephrotic syndrome or renal insufficiency the renal biopsy should be performed. Repeat kidney biopsies should also be done for clinical indications due to SLE flare, persistent proteinuria or declining renal function. The role of the renal biopsy in diagnosis, treatment, management, and follow-up of LN is critical, although to predict the outcome has been a matter of controversy [1, 7, 8]. Considering the importance of the biopsy making the treatment decision and determining the prognosis, it is essential to assess renal histopathology with high accuracy [9, 12, 13]. LN can affect all compartments of the kidney including glomeruli, tubules, interstitium and blood vessels. The analysis of the renal lesions is based on light microscopy (LM) associated with the immunofluorescence (IF) and electron microscopy (EM) findings [11].

3. Glomerular, tubulointerstitial and vascular lesions

The glomeruli are the most affected compartment in the LN. The initial injury is related to immune deposits in the mesangium and/or capillary loops. Large subendothelial deposits can be easily seen by LM. The distribution of deposits in the mesangium and/or glomerular capillaries defines the morphological pattern of the disease and consequently clinical manifestations. Some cases have only mesangial deposits, and others have deposits in the mesangium and in the capillary loops. Deposits in the capillary loops can be intramembranous, subendothelial (between endothelial cells and glomerular basement membrane) or subepithelial (between podocytes and glomerular basement membrane). Large subendothelial deposits characterize the wire loops and determine intense thickening of the glomerular basement membrane with occlusion of capillary loops (**Figure 1**). Immune deposits with complement activation determines an inflammatory reaction with proliferation of resident cells and exudation of mononuclear cells and polymorphonuclear neutrophils. Mesangial deposits stimulate proliferation of mesangial cells and deposition of mesangial matrix. Subendothelial deposits in capillary loops stimulate endothelial proliferation, and subepithelial deposits determines thickening of the GBM without significant cellular proliferation. Capillary involvement by the inflammatory response may result in segmental glomerular necrosis and adjacent cellular crescents. Prolonged glomerular injury result in segmental and/or global

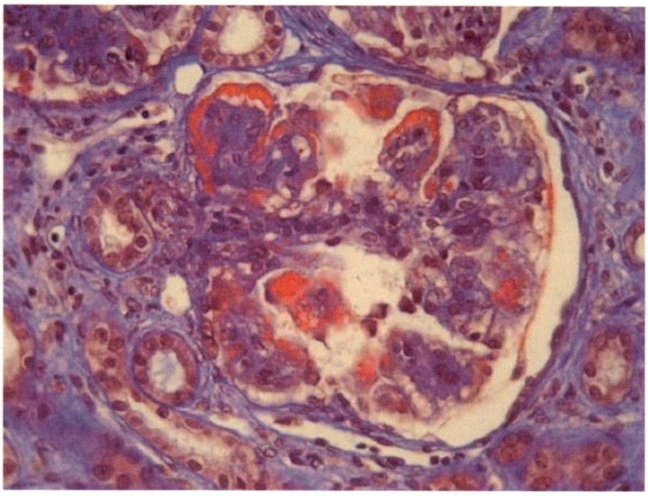

Figure 1.
Glomerulus with intense global hypercellularity and subendothelial hyaline deposits in peripheral capillary loops (wire loops). Masson thricrome 400x.

scarring. The IF staining is variable. IgG is the most frequent immunoglobulin (**Figure 2**), usually associated with deposits of C1q and C3. IgM and IgA deposits may also be present. Fibrin deposits are frequent in areas of necrosis and in association with active crescents. The IF staining is called the full house when there is deposition of the three immunoglobulins, C1q and C3. This staining pattern is very useful for diagnosing LN. The EM confirms the IF findings showing since small mesangial electron dense deposits to large and abundant deposits in the mesangium with extension to capillary loops. Immune deposits limited to the mesangium are associated with mild clinical signs and symptoms. The presence of deposits in the capillary loops, especially in the subendothelial space, is related to more harmful forms of the disease. Anti-dsDNA and anti-C1q antibodies correlate with

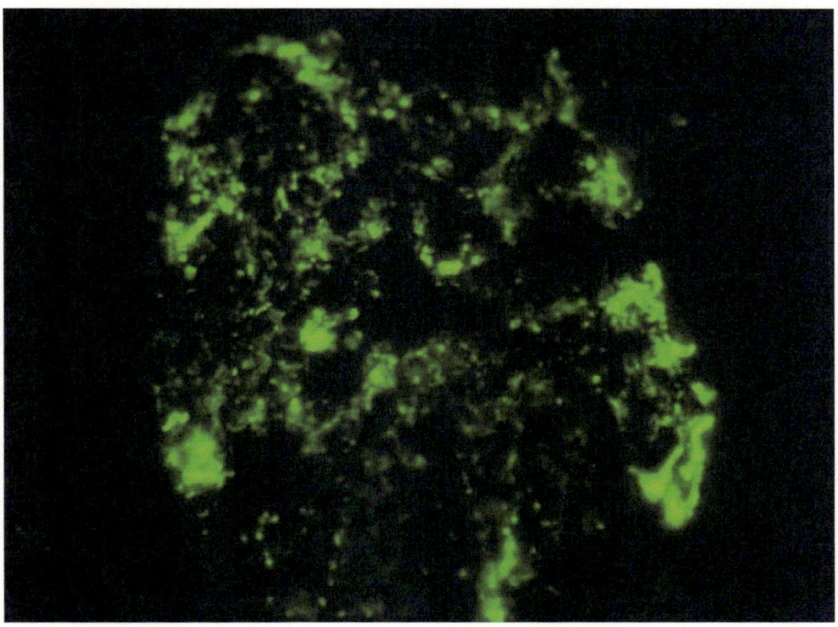

Figure 2.
Granular deposits of IgG in the mesangium and capillary loops. IF-400x.

subendothelial deposits that stimulate endothelial proliferation and glomerular necrosis. The most severe form of LN are cases of diffuse proliferative nephritis that show voluminous subendothelial deposits with high correlation with disease activity. Furthermore, during the course of the disease, LN can undergo transformations. Purely mesangial injuries can evolve to more severe mesangioendothelial proliferative disease with damage of capillary loops. After treatment, severe LN with endothelial proliferation can turn into mesangial proliferative lesion [7, 11].

Tubulointerstitial lesions are found in all types of glomerular lesions, although is more frequent in the most severe forms of proliferative LN. The lesions result from the autoimmune inflammatory activity of the disease and/or prolonged periods of proteinuria [11]. The acute phase is characterized by edema and inflammatory infiltrate with a predominance of mononuclear cells. Immune deposits are detected by IF and EM mainly in the tubular basement membrane and peritubular capillaries in 50% of the patients (**Figure 3**). Immunoglobulins are associated with complement components C1q and C3 in most cases. There was no correlation between prevalence of deposits and the severity of interstitial inflammation, suggesting that the immune complexes are not involved in the pathogenesis of interstitial nephritis in SLE [11, 14]. The predominance of T lymphocytes, CD4 or CD8, with frequent presence of monocytes and NK cells suggests cellular immunity. While several mechanisms may play an initial role, interstitial T cells and monocytes may be important determinants of pathogenesis of interstitial nephritis, and monocytes may be the major factor in the chronic injury and progression of LN [15]. On the other hand, nephrotic proteinuria also induces changes in the tubular cells due to active and excessive resorption of filtered proteins and lipoproteins by the proximal tubules [11]. After a prolonged period of damage, tubular atrophy and interstitial fibrosis characterize the chronic phase of the disease. Active and severe tubulointerstitial injury is most common in severe diffuse proliferative LN. The severity of interstitial inflammation correlated with the degree of renal insufficiency and was an accurate prognostic indicator of progressive deterioration of renal function. Many studies have shown an association between tubulointerstitial damage and a poor renal outcome in LN and in order to avoid progression to end

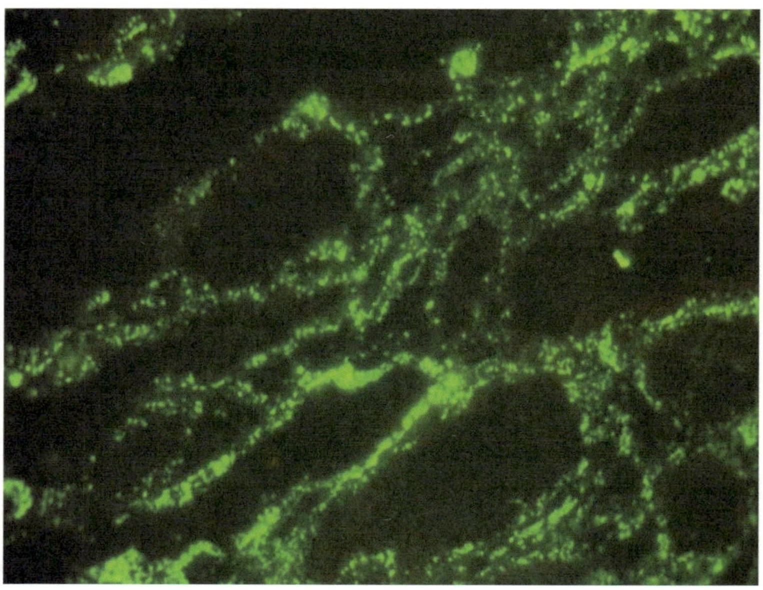

Figure 3.
Granular deposits of C1q in tubular basement membrane and peritubular spaces. IF-400x.

stage renal disease some studies suggest an early intervention before the development of interstitial fibrosis [15–18].

A variety of vascular lesions are encountered in renal biopsies of patients with SLE: uncomplicated vascular immune deposits, noninflammatory necrotizing vasculopathy, true renal vasculitis, thrombotic microangiopathy and arteriosclerosis. The interlobular arteries and arterioles are the most involved vessels [11, 19–21]. Large study with 285 patients with LN found vascular lesion in 79 (27.7%): 9.47% with noninflammatory necrotizing vasculopathy, 8.42% with thrombotic microangiopathy, 7.02% with arteriosclerosis and 2.81% with true vasculitis [20]. Wu *et al* [21] studying 341 patients with LN found 81.8% of vascular injury, including 74.19% of uncomplicated vascular immune deposits, 24.5% of arteriosclerosis, 17.59% of thrombotic microangiopathy, 3.81% of noninflammatory necrotizing vasculopathy and 0.59% of true vasculitis. The inclusion of cases of uncomplicated vascular immune deposits explains the higher incidence of vascular lesions in this study. Uncomplicated vascular immune deposits are the most common lesion and do not significantly affect prognosis. This type of injury shows deposits of immunoglobulins and complement in the small arteries and arterioles, without any inflammatory process and impairment of vascular lumen. The noninflammatory necrotizing vasculopathy determines severe vascular narrowing by abundant eosinophilic material constituted by immune deposits, plasma proteins and fibrin insudation in the vessel wall. There are also degenerative changes and loss of endothelial cells and myocytes. This is a form of vascular lesion associated to more severe forms of glomerular lesion, and is less common than uncomplicated vascular immune deposits. The necrotizing vasculopathy has a poor prognosis with a high degree of disease progression. A true renal vasculitis, with inflammatory infiltrate and necrosis of the vascular wall, is the least common vascular lesion in the LN. This kind of lesion is very severe with an ominous prognosis and need an aggressive immunosuppressive therapy. The thrombotic microangiopathy is characterized by myointimal proliferation of the small vessels, with a pattern of "onion skin", that complicates with thrombosis. In patients with SLE this vascular lesion occurs in association with hemolytic-uremic syndrome, antiphospholipid syndrome and malignant hypertension. Arteriosclerosis is a degenerative non-immunological vascular lesion characterized by fibrous thickening of the intima of the arteries without necrosis, proliferation or thrombosis. This lesion is common in LN due to the high prevalence of risk factors for arteriosclerosis in lupus patients such as hypertension, hyperlipidemia and prolonged use of corticosteroids. Vascular lesion can occur in any type of glomerular injury, but they are more frequent in the more active glomerulitis with mesangial and glomerular capillaries involvement [11, 19, 21]. Renal vascular lesions, specially of the necrotizing, vasculitic or thrombotic type adversely affects renal outcome with a higher rate of progression to renal failure [11, 19–21]. At the time of renal biopsy, patients with vascular lesion had higher levels of serum creatinine than patients without vascular lesion (2.2 mg/dl vs. 1.2 mg/dl). The probability of a kidney survival at 5 and 10 years was 74.3% and 58.0% in patients with vascular lesion, compared with 89.6% and 85.9% in patients without vascular lesion, respectively [20].

4. International Society of Nephrology and Renal Pathology Society Classification (2003)

The classifications of LN are based on glomerular morphologic lesions in different classes of LN and aim to identify patients at risk of progressing to chronic renal failure.

The morphological changes are based mainly under LM, although the combined analysis of IF and EM provide more effective study. The original World Health Organization (WHO) classification, formulated in 1974, defined 5 classes: Classes I-Normal glomeruli, II-Pure Mesangial Proliferation, III-Focal and segmental proliferative GN (<50% of glomeruli), IV-Diffuse Proliferative GN (≥50% of glomeruli) and V-Membranous GN. In 1995, the WHO classification was modified by the inclusion of subclasses enphasizing active and chronic lesions. However, the introduction of many subclasses has made it difficult to apply in practice. The subclasses of the membranous form of LN (class V) with proliferative lesions of class III (Vc) and class IV (Vd) were very controversial. The class V with additional proliferative features (Vc and Vd) showed a worse prognosis than pure class V, demonstrating that the prognosis was related to proliferative lesions and not to class V. These subcategories were eliminated, and instead, such complex lesions should be diagnosed as association of class V with classes III or IV [11]. The WHO classification has more recently evolved into the 2003 International Society of Nephrology and Renal Pathology Society classification (ISN/RPS) [22] (**Table 1**). The ISN/RPS nomenclature described only the immune-complex LN, not addressing other lesions such as thrombotic microangiopathy and podocytopathies. The ISN/RPS system classifies LN on the basis of where immune complexes accumulate in glomeruli, the presence or absence of mesangial or endocapillary proliferation, the overall extent of glomerular involvement (focal or diffuse; global or segmental) and whether glomerular injury is active (inflammatory) or chronic (sclerotic).

The schema ISN/RPS retains the major criteria of WHO classification with a revision and/or inclusion of pathologic details for each class. The "normal"category of the class I of WHO was eliminated, being replaced by the presence of mesangial deposits by IF and/or EM with normal LM. Class II besides deposits by IF or EM presents mesangial proliferation by LM. Classes III and IV present both mesangial and capillary deposits with endocapillary proliferation, and are separated based on the percentage of glomeruli affected by active and chronic lesions. The most

Classes	Type of Lesion
Class I-Mesangial LN	Normal LM, deposits IF or EM
Class II-Mesangial Proliferative LN	Mesangial hipercellularity and immune deposits by IF or EM
Class III-Focal LN III (A)-active lesions III (A/C)-active and chronic lesions III (C)-chronic lesions	< 50% glomeruli affected by segmental or global endo and/or extracapillary proliferation, subendothelial deposits, necrosis and crescents. Active and chronic lesions.
Class IV-Diffuse LN IV-S (A) or IV-G (A)-active lesions IV-S (A/C) or IV-G (A/C)-active and chronic lesions IV-S (C) or IV-G (C)-glomerular scars	≥50% glomeruli affected by segmental or global endo and/or extracapillary proliferation, subendothelial deposits, necrosis and crescents. Active and chronic lesions.
Class V-Membranous LN	Subepithelial deposits with thickening of GBM
Class VI-Advanced sclerosing LN	90% sclerosed glomeruli. Absence of residual activity.

Table 1.
International Society of Nephrology and Renal Pathology Society Classification of lupus Nephritis-2003 (ISN/RPS).

controversial aspect was the introduction of a subdivision of class IV based on whether the lesions are predominantly segmental or global [23]. Previous studies have suggested that a subgroup of LN with severe segmental lesions involving most of the glomeruli, may have a different pathogenesis than the global proliferative lesions of class III or IV. These severe segmental lesions often had necrosis and crescents, similar to pauci-immune necrotizing and crescentic GN. About 20% of patients with apparent necrotizing and crescentic LN, with rare or absent subendothelial deposits and without significant endocapillary proliferation, have positive ANCA suggesting a coexistence of LN and ANCA-associated necrotizing and crescentic GN [24]. Features of activity and chronicity was clearly delineated in the subcategories of class III and IV. Class IV has a higher risk of progression to chronic renal failure and large subendothelial deposits, necrosis and crescents have a worse prognosis. Due to the higher frequency of biopsied patients with more aggressive kidney injury, most series show a higher percentage of class IV [11]. The class VI was defined with glomerular sclerosis ≥90% of glomeruli without residual activity. Severe tubular atrophy, interstitial fibrosis, inflammation, and arteriosclerosis usually accompany the glomerular sclerosis. Chronic lesions, such as segmental or global sclerosis, are interpreted as sequelae of previous more aggressive lesions in the current classification. Thus, a segmentally sclerosing lesion producing an adhesion to Bowman's capsule, most likely represents an organization of a lesion with endothelial proliferation and/or necrosis and crescents, and should be interpreted as a chronic lesion of class III or IV. Globally sclerosed glomeruli can be particularly challenging, because ischemic collapse of the glomerular tuft with collagenous material in Bowman's space occur with aging and benign nephrosclerosis. This kind of lesion overlaps with sclerosed glomerulus with a fibrous crescent after an inflammatory process. Excess cells in the collagenous area, evidence of proliferative injury in the glomerular tuft with adhesion to the retracted and lamellate Bowman's capsule can help distinguish sclerosis due to LN from other causes of sclerosis [8].

Therefore, immune complex formation in the mesangium causes class I and II lesions, subendothelial deposits causes classes III and IV and subepithelial deposits occur in class V lesions.

5. Activity and chronicity indices

It has been known that immunosuppressive therapy is capable of reducing the amount of immune deposits and the degree of inflammatory process in the kidney. However, reduction of histological activity was not always accompanied by clinical improvement and, on the other hand, active lesions on the biopsy may be associated with a silent clinical presentation. These findings demonstrate the importance of renal biopsy in monitoring patients. Investigators have attempted to analyze renal biopsy specimens of LN with respect to active and chronic features as predictors of outcome and guides to therapy. Active lesions are potentially treatable and only the most severe ones become chronic, whereas chronic lesions represent irreversible damage with great impact in the outcome [25]. The concept of activity and chronicity indices was adopted in the studies of National Institutes of Health (NIH) (**Table 2**). According to this system, the activity (AI) and chronicity indices (CI) are graded on a scale of 0 to 24 and 0 to 12, respectively, by calculating the sum of individual scores (0 to 3+). In a group of patients with diffuse proliferative disease (Class IV), Austin *et al* [25] found that AI is moderately predictive of outcome, with 60% 10-year survival with AI greater than 12. Another study [26] showed 40% of impairment of renal function in 4 years with AI > 12 compared to 7% in the group with AI < 12. The CI was more predictive of renal outcome than

Indices	Grades
Activity Index (0–24)	
Endocapillary hypercellularity Subendothelial deposits Necrosis Cellular crescents	0 absent 1+ <25% of glomeruli 2+ 25–50% of glomeruli (x2) 3+ >50% of glomeruli (x2)
Leukocyte infiltration Interstitial inflammation	0 absent 1+ mild 2+ moderate 3+ severe
Chronicity Index (0–12)	
Glomerular sclerosis Fibrous crescents	0 absent 1+ <25% of glomeruli 2+ 25–50% of glomeruli 3+ >50% of glomeruli
Tubular atrophy Interstitial fibrosis	0 absent 1+ mild 2+ moderate 3+ severe

Table 2.
Activity and chronicity indices of lupus nephritis according to National Institutes of Health (NIH).

AI, demonstrating a 100% 10-year survival with CI ≤ 1, 68% with CI of 2 or 3 and 32% with CI ≥ 4. Although individual activity scores do not show predictive value for disease progression, all the scores of CI were individually predictive of renal failure, particularly tubular atrophy [25]. A combination of different scores also shows impact on the prognosis. There are a high risk of doubled creatinine with a combination of two scores, such as more than 50% of cellular crescents and moderate to severe interstitial fibrosis. Patients with severe disease treated with aggressive immunossuppression showed that AI > 7 and CI > 3 have a high risk of progression [27]. More than 5o% of crescents are a very ominous morpological finding, but even with <50% of crescents but combined with moderate or severe fibrosis the risk of doubled creatinine is high specially in black patients [28].

Renal biopsy does not adequately predict the progression of long-term lesions due to disagreement between signs of clinical and histological activity of the disease. Patients in clinical remission show in repeated biopsies evidence of active inflammatory process. On the other hand, in the absence of histological activity, cases of patients with persistent clinical signs are described. Thus, studies have suggested that serial biopsies during maintenance therapy may help in patient monitoring [7]. Alsuwaida *et al* [29] when analyzing a second renal biopsy at the end of the maintenance therapy, demonstrated that persistence of glomerular hypercellularity and interstitial inflammation presented a higher risk of doubling serum creatinine. Patients with an activity index greater than 2 in the second biopsy showed worse renal survival at 10 years and regarding the chronicity index there was a trend for better renal survival with a CI lower than 3.

6. Clinical findings and management

In order to prevent CKD, all patients with SLE should be evaluated for kidney involvement at initial diagnosis and at follow-up. Assessment of patients with suspected LN are greatly facilitated through information obtained by renal biopsy, and early diagnosis with response to therapy is correlated with better outcome [7, 9]. The heterogeneous morphological aspects of the disease is accompanied by a variable clinical findings. The different classes of LN guide clinicians in making the most appropriate therapeutic decision. A purely mesangial disease sparing the peripheral glomerular capillaries (classes I and II) usually have a mild disease with low levels of proteinuria and normal renal function. The prognosis is excellent and the patients require only conservative treatment. In many patients it is a stable lesion that may persist for years. However, it can undergo transformation to a more severe injury with increased levels of proteinuria and reduced kidney function [7]. LN with capillary loops injuries (classes III and IV) that shows more endocapillar proliferation, necrosis and crescents, with a coexistence of active and chronic lesions, have more aggressive disease. Tubular and interstitial lesions are nearly universal in diffuse proliferative LN and parallel the distribution of the glomerular lesions. Vascular lesions also occur most frequently in the diffuse proliferative group. The clinical manifestations are represented by high levels of proteinuria with or without nephrotic syndrome and active urinary sediment. In class III renal insufficiency is uncommon and the prognosis is variable. In a small percentage of patients there is poor outcome which results from progression of class III to class IV. The diffuse proliferative LN (class IV) have the most severe and active clinical renal presentation, with nephrotic syndrome in up 50% of the patients and various degrees of renal insufficiency in greater than 50% of the patients [30, 31]. It is a consensus that class IV has a worse prognosis. The proliferative classes with more severe active lesions (III and IV) are treated with potent immunosuppression [1, 8]. Some investigators proposed that class IV-S is pathogenetically distinct and has worse long-term outcome than class IV-G, suggesting important prognostic differences [23]. LN class IV-G has predominantly subendothelial deposits and endocapillary proliferation and patients with class IV-S much higher rate of segmental fibrinoid necrosis [32]. Segmental and global glomerulosclerosis are the consequence of active necrotizing lesions with crescent formation. The prognostic significance of class IV-S versus IV-G has been analyzed in other studies and no significant differences in outcome were demonstrated [32–34].

All patients with class V LN have proteinuria and 59–70% have the nephrotic syndrome. Renal insufficiency is uncommon. Patients with class V are more likely to present with renal disease before other systemic features of lupus are apparent. When a membranous lesion is associated with the active or chronic lesions of class III or IV, both diagnoses are to be reported. Patients with membranous LN (class V) may be managed conservatively with antiproteinuric therapy when proteinuria is subnephrotic or with immunosuppression with nephrotic proteinuria [7]. Patients with class VI lupus nephritis have severe renal insufficiency and require only supportive treatment and/or kidney replacement therapy [7].

7. Controversial aspects of ISN/RPS classification and NIH activity and chronicity indices

The classification of INS/RPS was proposed to standardize and emphasize the most relevant lesions to guide the treatment of LN. Recently, several retrospective validation studies concerning the utility of the classification were performed. These studies have highlighted the limitations of the classification and of the activity and chronicity indices. In these reports, the main weaknesses of the classification include: 1. Tubulointerstitial and vascular lesions not included in the system; 2. No correlation between the lesions with long-term outcome; 3. Poor interobserver reproducibility of both active and chronic lesions [12, 13, 32–35].

Tubulointerstitial and vascular lesions correlated closely with clinical disease activity and renal outcome in many studies [14, 19–21]. It is necessary at least to mention these lesions in the diagnosis of the biopsy report.

The classification of LN, especially classes IV-G and IV-S, and the activity and chronicity indexes have not shown a satisfactory correlation with the long-term outcome of the disease [1, 7, 8, 13]. After treatment induction and even during the maintenance phase, the inflammatory process may persist and go unnoticed clinically. Some authors recommend repeating the renal biopsy after treatment to better assess the response to treatment and predict the course of the disease [1, 7, 8, 29]. There is also a poor reproducibility among pathologists to apply these criteria that limits their application in practice [1, 36, 37]. It is a consensus that the classification of LN as well as the criteria of activity and chronicity of the disease should be reviewed [1, 7, 8, 36, 37].

8. Conclusions

In conclusion, the precise identification of key glomerular, tubulointerstitial and vascular lesions remain incompletely understood in terms of pathogenesis and prognostic effect. The ISN/RPS classification improved the knowledge of different patterns of LN lesions, and validation studies have shown new emerging morphological data to be further investigated and included in the classification [8, 12, 35]. Most nephrologists find an assessment of activity and chronicity

Biopsy Report

ID: RPS, caucasian, female with 38 years-old

History: Patient with erythema and scaling in the face, lymphocitopenia, anemia, proteinuria of 2g/24h, microhematuria, serum creatinine of 1,8 mg/dl. Anti-dsDNA>200 UI, ANA 1/1600.

Renal biopsy

Macroscopy: 3 fragments of renal biopsy measuring each 1cm long. One fragment fixated in Duboscq-Brazil was sent to LM, 1 frozen fragment was sent to IF using anti-IgG, IgA, IgM, C1q, C3, Fibrin, κ and λ conjugates, 1 fixated in glutaraldehyde 2,5% sent to EM.

Light Microscopy: Renal biopsy showing the cortical with 30 glomeruli, all with large size and mesangioendothelial heavy hypercellularity and moderate exsudate of polymorphonuclear neutrophils; some peripheral capillary loops show bulky hyaline deposits obliterating capillary lumens (wire loops). In 6 glomeruli there are small segments fibrinoid necrosis, nuclear debris and fibrin deposits, with overlying small cellular crescents. Two glomeruli are globally sclerosed surrounded by tubular atrophy and mild interstitial fibrosis. There is also a heavy interstitial edema and inflammatory infiltrate of mononuclear cells with degenerative changes of tubules. The vessels are unremarkable.

Immunofluorescence: Presence of diffuse granular deposits in the mesangium and capillary loops of IgG (3/3+), IgA (2/3+), IgM (1/3+), C1q (3/3+), C3 (2/3+), Fibrin (2/3+), κ and λ (2/3+). There were deposits in the tubular basement membrane and peritubular capillaries of IgG and C1q (2/3+). There were no deposits in the vessels.

Electron microscopy: Presence of mesangial, subendothelial and tubular basement membrane electron-dense deposits.

Renal biopsy diagnosis: Lupus nephritis characterized by diffuse proliferative glomerulonephritis with 20% of segmental necrosis, 20% of cellular crescents and 6,6% of global glomerular sclerosis. Intense lymphomononuclear tubulointerstitial nephritis with focal tubular atrophy and interstitial fibrosis. Normal vessels.

ISN/RPS classification: Class IV-G (A/C)

NIH Activity and Chronicity Indices:

Activity: subendothelial deposits 2+, glomerular hypercellularity 3+, exsudate of neutrophils 2+, necrosis 2+, cellular crescents 2+, interstitial inflammatory infiltrate 3+. Total = 14

Chronicity: glomerular sclerosis 1+, tubular atrophy 1+, interstitial fibrosis 1+. Total =3

Box 1.
Biopsy Report Interpretation of Lupus Nephritis

indices useful, and the biopsy reports should include routinely, with a detailed description of the types of active and chronic lesions and proportion of glomeruli affected (**Figures 1–3** and **Box 1**). Despite these unresolved controversies, active lesions versus chronic lesions, in addition to class of LN, influence response to therapy. The ISN/RPS recently presented a consensus report from a meeting of an international nephropathology working group in 2016. Briefly, they proposed new definitions for mesangial hypercellularity and different patterns of crescents; endocapillary proliferation was replaced by endocapillary hypercellularity, the IV-S and IV-G subclasses were eliminated, and active and chronic designations of class III and IV were replaced by the activity and chronicity indices that should be applied to all classes. In order to improve the LN classification, further studies will be carried out to validate the new proposal [38].

Acknowledgements

We thank our professors, the Department of Pathology and the Botucatu Medical School for all the learning that allowed this work.

Conflict of interest

The authors declare no conflict of interest.

Author details

Rosa Marlene Viero* and Daniela Cristina dos Santos
Department of Pathology, Botucatu Medical School, UNESP, Botucatu, SP, Brazil

*Address all correspondence to: rosa.viero@unesp.br

References

[1] Parikh SV, Almaani S, Brodsky S, Rovin BH. Update on Lupus Nephritis: Core Curriculum 2020. AJKD 2020; 76 (2): 265-281.

[2] Worrall JG, Snaith ML, Batchelor JR, Isenberg DA. SLE: a rheumatological view. Analysis of the clinical features, serology and immunogenetics of 100 SLE patients during long-term follow-up. Q J Med 1990; 74 (275): 319-330.

[3] Malafronte P, Mastroianni-Kirsztajn G, Betônico G, Romão Jr JE, Alves MAR, Carvalho MF, Viera Neto OM, Cadaval RAM, Bérgamo RR, Woronik V, Sens YAS, Marrocos MSM, Barros RT. Paulista registry of glomerulonephritis: 5-year data report. Nephrol Dial Transplant 2006; 21: 3098-3105.

[4] Rivera F, Lopez-Gomez JM, Perez-Garcia R. Spanish Registry of Glomerulonephritis. Frequency of renal pathology in Spain 1994-1999. Nephrol Dial Transplant 2002; 17: 1594-1602.

[5] Li LS, Liu ZH. Epidemiologic data of renal diseases from a single unit in China: analysis based on 13.519 renal biopsies. Kidney Int 2004; 66: 920-923.

[6] Borchers AT, Keen CL, Shoenfeld Y, Gershuin ME. Surviving the butterfly and the wolf: mortality trends in systemic lupus erythematosus. Autoimmunity Reviews 2004; 3:423-453.

[7] Almaani S, Meara A, Rovin BH. Update on Lupus Nephritis. Clin J Am Soc Nephrol 2017; 12 (5): 825-835.

[8] Giannico G, Fogo AB. Lupus Nephritis: Is the Kidney Biopsy Currently Necessary in the Management of Lupus Nephritis? Clin J Am Soc Nephrol 2013; 8: 138-145.

[9] Satish S, Deka P, Shetty MS. A clinico-pathological study of lupus nephritis based on the International Society of Nephrology-Renal Pathology Society 2003 classification system. J Lab Phys 2017; 9 (3): 149-155.

[10] Tan EM, Cohen AS, Fries JF, Masi AT, McShane DJ, Rothfield NF, Schaller JG, Talal N, Winchester RJ. The 1982 revised criteria for the classification of systemic lupus erythematosus. Arthritis Rheum 1982; 25 (11): 1271-1277.

[11] D'Agati VD, Stokes MB. Renal disease in systemic lupus erythe matosus, mixed connective tissue disease, Sjögren syndrome, and rheumatoid arthritis. In: Jennette JC, Olson JL, Silva FG, D'Agati VD, editors. Hepinstall's Pathology of Kidney. 7th Ed. Philadelphia-PA, USA: Wolters Kluwer; 2015. p. 559-656.

[12] Dasari S, Chakraborty A, Truong L, Mohan C. A Systematic Review of Interpathologist Agreement in Histologic Classification of Lupus Nephritis. Kidney Int Rep 2019; 4: 1420-1425.

[13] Sada KE, Makino H. Usefulness of ISN/RPS Classification of Lupus Nephritis. J Korean Med Sci 2009; 24 (Suppl 1): S7-10.

[14] Park MH, D'Agati VD, Appel GB, Pirani CL. Tubulointerstitial disease in lupus nephritis: relationship to immune deposits, interstitial inflammation, glomerular changes, renal function, and prognosis. Nephron 1986; 44: 309-319.

[15] Alexopoulos E, Seron D, Hartley RB, Cameron JS. Lupus nephritis: correlation of interstitial cells with glomerular function. Kidney Int 1990; 37 (1): 100-109.

[16] Broder A, Mowrey WB, Khan HN, Jovanovic B, Londono-jimenez A, Izmirly P, Putterman C. Tubulo interstitial Damage Predicts End Stage Renal Disease in Lupus Nephritis with Preserved to Moderately Impaired Renal Function: a Retrospective Cohort Study. Semin Arthritis Rheum 2018; 47(4): 545-551.

[17] Clark MR, Trotter K, Chang A. The pathogenesis and therapeutic implications of tubulointerstitial inflammation in human lupus nephritis. Semin Nephrol 2015; 35(5): 455-464.

[18] Jimenez AL, Mowrey WB, Putterman C, Buyon J, Goilav B, Broder A. Tubulointerstitial Damage in Lupus Nephritis: A Comparison of the Factors Associated with Tubulo interstitial Inflammation and Renal Scarring. Arthritis Rheumatol. 2018; 70(11): 1801-1806.

[19] Appel GB, Pirani CL, D'Agati V: Renal vascular complications of systemic lupus erythematosus. J Am Soc Nephrol 1994; 4: 1499-1515.

[20] Banfi G, Bertani T, Boeri V, Faraggiana T, Mazzucco G, Monga G, Sacchi G. Renal vascular lesions as a marker of poor prognosis in patients with lupus nephritis. Gruppo Italiano per lo Studio della Nefrite Lupica (GISNEL). Am J Kidney Dis 1991; 18 (2): 240-248.

[21] Wu LH, Yu F, Tan Y, Qu Z, Chen MH, Wang SX, Liu G, Zhao MH. Inclusion of renal vascular lesions in the 2003 ISN/RPS system for classifying lupus nephritis improves renal outcome predictions. Kidney Int 2013; 83: 715-723.

[22] Weening JJ, D'Agati VD, Schwartz MM, Seshan SV, Alpers CE, Appel GB, Balow JE, Bruijn JA, Cook T, Ferrario F, Fogo AB, Ginzler EM, Hebert L, Hill G, Hill P, Jennette JC, Kong NC, Lesavre P, Lockshin M, Looi LM, Makino H, Moura LA, Nagata M. The Classification of Glomerulonephritis in Systemic Lupus Erythematosus Revisited. J Am Soc Nephrol 2004; 15: 241-250.

[23] Najafi CC, Korbet SM, Lewis EJ, Schwartz MM, Reichlin M, Evans J; Lupus Nephritis Collaborative Study Group: Significance of histologic patterns of glomerular injury upon long-term prognosis in severe lupus glomerulonephritis. Kidney Int 2001; 59: 2156-2163.

[24] Nasr SH, D'Agati VD, Park HR, Sterman PL, Goyzueta JD, Dressler RM, Hazlett SM, Pursell RN, Caputo C, Markowitz GS: Necrotizing and crescentic lupus nephritis with antineutrophil cytoplasmic antibody seropositivity. Clin J Am Soc Nephrol 2008; 3: 682-690.

[25] Austin III HA, Muenz LR, Joyce KM, Antonovych TA, Kullick ME, Klippel JH, Decker JL, Balow JE. Prognostic factors in lupus nephritis. Contribution of renal histologic data. Am J Med 1983; 75 (3):382-391.

[26] Austin III HA, Muenz LR, Joyce KM, Antonovych TT, Balow JE. Diffuse proliferative lupus nephritis: identification of specific pathologic features affecting renal outcome. Kidney Int 1984; 25 (4): 689-695.

[27] Austin III HA, Boumpas DT, Vaughan EM, Balow JE. Predicting renal outcomes in severe lupus nephritis: contributions of clinical and histological data. Kidney Int 1994; 45 (2): 544-550.

[28] Austin III HA, Boumpas DT, Vaughan EM, Balow. High-risk features of lupus nephritis: importance of race and clinical and histological factors in 166 patients. Nephrol Dial Transplant 1995; 10: 1620-1628.

[29] Alsuwaida A, Husain S, Alghonaim M, AlOudah N, Alwakeel J,

ullah A, Kfoury H: Strategy for second kidney biopsy in patients with lupus nephritis. Nephrol Dial Transplant 2012; 27: 1472-1478.

[30] Appel GB, Silva FG, Pirani CL, Meltzer JI, Estes D. renal involvement in systemic lupus erithematosus (SLE): a study of 56 patients emphasinzing histologic classification. Medicine (Baltimore) 1978; 57: 371.

[31] Baldwin DS, Gluck MC, Lowenstein J, Gallo GR. Lupus nephritis: clinical course as related to morphologic forms and their transitions. Am J Med 1977; 62:12-30.

[32] Hill GS, Delahousse M, Nochy D, Bariety J. Class IV-S versus class IV-G lupus nephritis: clinical and morphologic differences suggesting different pathogenesis. Kidney Int 2005; 68: 2288-2297.

[33] Mittal B, Hurwitz S, Rennke H, Singh AK: New subcategories of class IV lupus nephritis: Are there clinical, histologic, and outcome differences? Am J Kidney Dis 2004; 44: 1050-1059.

[34] Yu F, Tan Y, Wu LH, Zhu SN, Liu G, Zhao MH: Class IV-G and IV-S lupus nephritis in Chinese patients: A large cohort study from a single center. Lupus 2009; 18: 1073-1081.

[35] Mubarak M, Nasri H. ISN/RPS 2003 classification of lupus nephritis: time to take a look on the achievements and limitations of the schema. J Nephropathol. 2014; 3(3): 87-90.

[36] Schwartz MM, Lan SP, Bernstein J, Hill GS, Holley K, Lewis EJ. Role of pathology indices in the management of severe lupus glomerulonephritis. Lupus Nephritis Collaborative Study Group. Kidney Int 1992; 42 (3): 743-748.

[37] Schwartz MM, Lan SP, Bernstein J, Hill GS, Holley K, Lewis EJ. Irreproducibility of the activity and chronicity indices limits their utility in the management of lupus nephritis. Lupus Nephritis Collaborative Study Group. Am J Kidney Dis 1993; 21 (4): 374-377.

[38] Bajema IM, Wilhelmus S, Alpers CE, Bruijn JA, Colvin RB, Cook HT, D'Agati VD, Ferrario F, Haas M, Jennette JC, Joh K, Nast CC, Nöel LH, Rijnink EC, Roberts ISD, Seshan SV, Sethi S, Fogo AB. Revision of the International Society of Nephrology/ Renal Pathology Society classification for lupus nephritis: clarification of definitions, and modified National Institutes of Health activity and chronicity indices. Kidney Int 2018; 93, 789-796.

Chapter 3

Lupus Nephritis: Current Updates

Fahd Adeeb and Wan Ahmad Hafiz Wan Md Adnan

Abstract

Lupus is a heterogenous multisystem autoimmune disease whereby nephritis is one of its most common cause of overall morbidity and mortality. Accurate, timely diagnosis and effective treatment in lupus nephritis (LN) remains a challenge to many clinicians including those who are directly involved in the daily care of these patients. Despite significant improvement in patients' survival rate in recent years, in this era of precision medicine, there is pressing need to further improve our understanding and management of this disease. Our chapter would shed light on the key issues in LN including recent advances in our scientific understanding of its' pathophysiology, major challenges and treatment strategies.

Keywords: SLE, lupus, nephritis

1. Introduction

Lupus nephritis (LN) is the most common severe organ manifestation of systemic lupus erythematosus (SLE). It may be the presenting manifestation of SLE and usually arises within 5 years of diagnosis [1]. Approximately 40–70% of SLE patients will develop LN [2] with histopathological changes observed in most patients even among those without renal manifestations (known as "silent LN"; mostly with "milder" class I and II histologic lesions) [3, 4]. Clinical presentation of LN is highly variable, ranging from asymptomatic proteinuria with normal renal function to rapidly progressive renal failure.

Recent data demonstrates reduction in the temporal mortality trend among end stage renal disease (ESRD) LN patients [5]; however, the risk of progression to ESRD in LN remains unchanged [5, 6]. Despite significant improvement of outcome in this modern era, less than 50% of patients achieve complete clinical remission following immune suppression [7] with 10–20% of patients progressing to ESRD [8]. This chapter explores recent studies that have substantially contributed to our understanding of LN and provides new insights into the epidemiology, pathogenesis, classification criteria and management strategies of LN.

2. Epidemiology

The prevalence of SLE and LN varies based on age, gender, geographical location, socioeconomic status and ethnicity. There are also disproportionate differences in the incidence and prevalence, depending upon the validated classification criteria or methods of case ascertainment used.

2.1 Systemic lupus erythematosus (SLE)

In a large retrospective study performed in the United Kingdom (UK) involving more than 7,000 SLE cases between 1999 and 2012, the overall annual incidence of SLE was 4.9 cases per 100,000 population per year with overall prevalence of 97 per 100,000 population; highest in Afro-Caribbean ethnic subgroup (517 per 100,000), followed by the Indian subgroup (193 per 100,000) while Caucasian subgroup was 134 per 100,000 [9]. Other studies found similar estimates with annual incidence between 4 and 8 cases per 100,000 population per year. Expectedly, the worldwide prevalence of SLE also varies between 30 to 90 cases per 100,000 population, highest in the African populations, lowest in Caucasians, with Hispanic and Asian subgroups in between the two extremes [10, 11].

All studies worldwide have demonstrated marked predominance of women in SLE, between 6 and 9 times higher than men. In the United States (US) and UK, the peak incidence was in women aged between 40 and 59 [10, 12]; in contrast, a population based study in Taiwan involving almost 7000 SLE patients revealed earlier peak incidence in women aged between 20 and 29 [13], a consistent trend among other studies in the Asia-Pacific region [14].

2.2 Lupus nephritis (LN)

Renal involvement occurs in 25–50% of SLE patients at the time of diagnosis [15]. The cumulative incidence, again, varies according to ethnicities. In a US study involving three ethnic subgroups, the incidence of LN was found to be the highest among the African subgroup (69%) followed by Hispanics (61%) and Caucasians (29%) [16]. In the Asia-Pacific region, the cumulative incidence of LN varies between 30% and 82%, lowest in Australian and highest in Malaysian populations respectively [14].

Despite higher overall incidence of SLE in women than in men, strikingly, renal involvement was found to be 50% higher in SLE men in a meta-analysis involving nearly 12,000 SLE patients across multiple countries [17]. Left untreated, LN carries significant morbidity and mortality, with the mortality rate estimated to be 6 times higher than general population. However, with the current therapeutic options, the 10-year survival for patients with LN can exceed 98% [18].

3. Pathogenesis

The pathogenesis of LN is complex and achieving full understanding of its pathophysiologic mechanisms has proved challenging due to the molecular and phenotypic heterogeneity. Genetic predisposition, epigenetic dysregulation and environmental triggers are all likely to contribute to the disease expression [1, 19, 20]. Dysregulation of both innate and adaptive immune responses manifested by disturbance in apoptotic cell clearance, cytokines stimulation, B-cell immunity and T-cell function leads to glomerular and/or tubulointerstitial injury.

Production of autoantibodies targeting self-DNA, other self-nuclear antigens and non-nuclear materials results from loss of immune self-tolerance and autoimmunity in genetically predisposed individuals. Formation of immune complexes (ICs) may occur in circulation and deposits in various organ systems including the kidneys. Antibodies can also directly target in situ nephritogenic antigens at the major resident renal cells (mesangial cells, glomerular endothelial cells, tubular epithelial cells and podocytes) [21]. Co-stimulation by Fc receptors (FcRs) and endosomal Toll-like receptors (TLRs) leads to activation of the complement system and subsequent release of cytokines and chemokines leading to renal tissue injury [22–25]. Anti-C1q antibodies, while not exclusive to LN, are strongly associated with renal inflammation and severe LN, amplifying complement activation in situ [26, 27].

Overactivation of 1) Interferon (IFN)-I signalling pathway, which is regulated by dendritic cells (DCs), interleukins (eg. IL 12/23), JAK1, TYK2 and various STAT proteins and 2) NFκB are both implicated early in the innate immune response and play major roles in the pathogenesis [28, 29]. Adaptive responses including persistent activation and interaction of aberrant polyclonal B and T cells involving multiple co-stimulatory molecules promote chronic inflammation and renal tissue damage. Studies have also uncovered that formation of long-lived memory T-cells and plasma cells that reside in survival niches in bone marrow and inflamed tissue render them resistant to conventional immunosuppression or B cell therapies [30].

B cell activation factor (BAFF)/B-lymphocyte stimulator (BLyS) promotes formation of tertiary lymphoid structures (TLSs) that contribute to lymphocyte priming and autoantibody production within the kidneys [31] while evidence in patients and animal models have demonstrated high levels of IL-17 producing T cells in LN [32]. Several other regulators of apoptosis have also been implicated in the development of LN including dysregulation of autophagy, BCL-2, phosphatase and tensin homologue (PTEN), mannose-binding lectin (MBL) and neutrophil extracellular traps (NETs) among several others [33–40].

More than 10 genome-wide association studies (GWAS) have been conducted thus far with more than 50 genes implicated involving various pathogenic mechanisms in the pathogenesis of SLE, some associated with LN [2, 41]. These candidate genes are likely to undergo further evaluation and validation from deep sequencing and mechanistic studies. *Mohan et al.* have elegantly categorised the implicated genes into four functional groups; genes that influence 1) lymphocyte activation, particularly B cells (eg. BLK, STAT4, TNFSF4, HLA-DR) 2) innate immune signalling (notably NFκB and IFN-I; eg. IKZF1, IRF5, TLR9, TNFAIP3) 3) intra-renal signalling (eg. ACE, KLK) and 4) handling of apoptotic material, chromatin and ICs (eg. ATG5, ITGAM, FCGR2A/3A/3B); genetic interaction from multiple categories is required for severe LN to develop [2].

The TLR7 gene, which is located at chromosome X, has recently been the focus of considerable research in SLE and LN. Theories regarding the contribution of TLR7 gene have included 1) Enhanced TLR7 protein expression in renal DCs and macrophages which correlated with renal disease parameters in murine models [42] 2) Emerging evidence that TLR7 dosage is a key pathogenic factor to the pathogenesis of SLE: *Dillon et al.* assembled the largest group consisting of 316 men with SLE and found high prevalence of SLE in X chromosome aneuploides such as Klinefelter's syndrome (KS; 47, XXY) and de la Chapelle's syndrome (46, XX male) [43] while recently, Souyris and colleagues provided proof that TLR7gene evades X chromosome inactivation in immune cells in women and KS men, and proposed this as a mechanism for the elevated risk of SLE in women and KS [44], which may partially explain the high preponderance of SLE in females.

4. Diagnosis and classification

Current non-invasive SLE biomarkers such as proteinuria or active urine sediment, serum creatinine, anti dsDNA and hypocomplementemia could not reliably confirm the presence, severity and/or chronicity, or predict the outcome of LN. Many novel biomarkers are currently being explored in the management and as therapeutic target in LN; unfortunately, none so far had been utilised in daily clinical practice [45].

In patients suspected of LN, certain clinical and laboratory features may however predict the class of LN a patient may have. In a retrospective study analysing 297 renal biopsies of SLE patients with some degree of proteinuria, absence of malar rash, negative anti-dsDNA and urine leukocytes of <5/high power field under microscopy are independent predictors for class II LN. Class III or IV can independently be predicted by younger age at diagnosis (<32 years), musculoskeletal involvement, hypertension, presence of anti-dsDNA, elevated creatinine level, absence of nephrotic range proteinuria and presence of leucocytes and cellular cast in urine. Older age, malar rash and low C3 level may be predictive for class V LN [46].

4.1 Role of renal biopsy

Renal biopsy is the gold standard for the diagnosis and current classification of LN. The histological findings may assist physicians to optimise therapeutic strategies in individual patients, including assessing disease activity and/or chronicity for guidance to escalate or de-escalate immunosuppression accordingly. It is an invasive procedure with potential risks, most notably bleeding; however, given the lack of available biomarkers to identify disease activity, it remains an irreplaceable tool and mainstay of current management in LN.

Indication for a renal biopsy includes significant proteinuria of >0.5 g/day (or equivalent), certain unclear acute elevation of serum creatinine level, and in patients with severe disease relapse (**Table 1**) [47]. Biopsy is rarely done in patients with isolated haematuria or proteinuria of <0.5 g/day; hence, class I LN is rarely seen in the histology. Performed by either experienced nephrologist or interventional radiologist, adequate tissue is obtained in >95% of times.

Given the location of kidney where no direct compression can be performed post biopsy, bleeding (as detected by routine CT scan or ultrasound post biopsy) was found to be common, ranging in 57–91% of patients [48]; however, the actual incidence of clinically important bleeding is small. Meta-analysis of 34 relevant studies found low rates of macroscopic haematuria (3.5%) and blood transfusion (0.9%), with lower rates yielded in need for interventions (0.6%) such as catheter insertion for bladder obstruction (0.3%) and nephrectomy (0.01%) and death (0.02%) [49].

The bleeding risk increases in females, use of larger needle (14-G), elevated serum creatinine (>176 umol/L) or acute renal failure, uncontrolled systolic blood pressure (>170 mmHg) [49, 50] and in patients with coagulopathies or are on anticoagulation/antiplatelet agents. Most serious complications are detected within 4 hours of biopsy, and majority within 12 hours [51, 52]. Routine 1-hour post biopsy ultrasound for presence of haematoma to predict complication has not been shown to be clinically beneficial (positive predictive value of 43%; negative predictive value of 95%) [53].

Should biopsy	May biopsy
Proteinuria >0.5 g/24 hours	Isolated haematuria or pyuria
Unexplained renal insufficiency	Proteinuria less than 0.5 g/24 hours
Differentiating activity vs. chronicity	'Protocol' biopsy during/after treatment
Severe relapse	Mild relapse

Table 1.
Possible indications for kidney biopsy in SLE patient.

The role of repeat renal biopsy in LN flares is controversial. In essence, a repeat biopsy is required if it may change management; for example, this is particularly true in a patient with stable renal function who developed sudden deterioration of creatinine associated with active urine sediment. This may reflect the possibility of crescentic glomerulonephritis (GN) that warrants stronger immunosuppression. During LN flare, histological transformation is more likely to occur if the initial histology revealed non-proliferative disease (initial class II); although, many would still have persistent active lesions in proliferative disease [54, 55].

Renal biopsy may also be considered to determine disease chronicity in patients with persistent proteinuria and lower glomerular filtration rate (GFR), which warrant de-escalation of immunosuppression. It is well documented that repeat biopsies lead to change to immunosuppression in more than half of the cases [55].

Decision to stop maintenance immunosuppression in LN is often challenging and some researchers perform 'protocol biopsies' after a period of complete clinical remission to guide withdrawal of treatment. Its' value however is still debatable, as studies mostly looked at the prognosis based on the histological features [54]. In a study by *De Rosa et al.*, 36 LN patients on immunosuppressive therapy for more than 3 years and in clinical remission (proteinuria <0.5 g/day) were re-biopsied. Regardless of the results of biopsy, the immunosuppressive medications were tapered down. Those patients with residual activity in histology had higher chance of relapses upon reducing therapy [56], which supports histology-based approach in treatment withdrawal.

4.2 Classification criteria

4.2.1 SLE and renal involvement

The revised American College of Rheumatology (ACR) 1997 criteria specifies that a patient can be diagnosed with SLE if 4 of 11 criteria are met at any interval of observation (**Table 2**). Renal involvement can be considered if patient developed proteinuria of >0.5/day or appearance of cellular cast (red cells, haemoglobin, granular, tubular or mixed) [57]. The 2012 Systemic Lupus International Collaborating Clinics (SLICC) criteria divided SLE features into 11 clinical and 6 immunologic criteria, where SLE can be fulfilled by a) biopsy-proven LN in presence of ANA or anti-DNA antibodies or b) meeting ≥4 of 17 criteria, with at least 1 criterion from each division [58].

European League Against Rheumatism (EULAR)/ACR published a new set of criteria for SLE diagnosis in 2019 [58]. It employs the strategy that ANA must be positive for the diagnosis to be considered, followed by 10 domains with different individual weightage; diagnosis can be made if total score reaches 10 points, again with renal involvement carrying a high weight between 4 and 10 depending on the renal manifestations (**Table 2**) [59].

4.3 Diagnosis of lupus nephritis

The clinical presentations of LN may differ ranging from asymptomatic haematuria to rapidly progressive GN. All patients with SLE should have urinalysis checked on regular basis to detect renal involvement. Presence of significant proteinuria would trigger the need for a renal biopsy, although many would perform biopsies for reasons such as persistent haematuria and elevated serum creatinine [54]. Biopsy is critical to distinguish between active nephritis, non-glomerular pathology of SLE (such as tubulointerstitial nephritis or thrombotic microangiopathy) and disease chronicity (such as interstitial fibrosis, tubular atrophy and

ACR 1997	**SLICC 2012**	**ACR 2019**
4 out of 11 criteria	4 out of 17 criteria, with at least 1 from each domain	Fulfil the entry criterion, followed by 10 points in additive criteria
Malar rash	**Clinical Domain**	**Entry criterion**
Discoid rash	Acute cutaneous lupus	ANA positive
Photosensitivity	Chronic cutaneous lupus	**Additive criteria**
Oral ulcer	Oral ulcer	**Clinical domain**
Arthritis	Synovitis	Constitutional
Serositis	Non-scarring alopecia	*Fever* (2)
Renal disease	Serositis	Haematologic
Neurologic disorder	Renal	*Leukopenia* (3)
Haematologic disorder	Neurologic	*Thrombocytopenia* (4)
Immunologic disorder	Haemolytic anaemia	*Autoimmune haemolysis* (4)
ANA positive	Leukopenia or lymphopenia	Neuropsychiatric
	Thrombocytopenia	*Delirium* (2)
	Immunologic Domain	*Psychosis* (3)
	ANA	*Seizure* (5)
	Anti dsDNA	Mucocutaneous
	Anti-Sm	*Non-scarring alopecia* (2)
	Antiphospholipid antibody	*Oral ulcers* (2)
	Low complement	*Subcutanoues OR discoid lupus* (4)
	Direct Coomb's test	*Acute cutaneous lupus* (6)
		Serosal
		Pleural/Pericardial effusion (5)
		Acute pericarditis (6)
		Musculoskeletal
		Joint involvement (6)
		Renal
		Proteinuria > 0.5 g/24 h (4)
		Renal biopsy class II or V (8)
		Renal biopsy class III or IV (10)
		Immunology domain
		Antiphospholipid antibodies
		Anti-cardiolipin OR
		anti-B2GP1 antibodies OR
		lupus anticoagulant (2)
		Complement proteins
		Low C3 OR low C4 (3)
		Low C3 AND low C4 (4)
		SLE-specific antibodies
		Anti-dsDNA antibody OR
		anti-Smith antibody (6)

Table 2.
Criteria for SLE diagnosis based on different criteria.

glomerulosclerosis). Importantly, biopsy findings should be interpreted and correlated carefully with patients' clinical features and serology.

In an analysis by *Ishizaki et al.* of 48 SLE patients who had renal biopsies but no urine abnormality, 36 patients were identified to have some morphologic changes. Although majority had class I/II (72%), six (17%) patients were found to have class III/IV LN [60]. LN has characteristic histological features that differ from other glomerular pathology and may involve lesions in the glomerular, vascular or tubulointerstitial structures. Analysis of 860 renal biopsies by *Kudose S et al.* confirmed 5 histopathological features of LN; 1) "full-house" staining by immunofluorescence (IF) 2) intense C1q staining 3) extraglomerular deposits 4) combined subendothelial and subepithelial deposits and 5) endothelial tubuloreticular inclusion [61].

The first published classification of glomerular changes in LN was formulated in 1974 under the auspices of the World Health Organisation (WHO; **Table 3**). It divides glomerular changes into five classes, which became the basis of today's classification. Class I applies to biopsies with no detectable changes in glomeruli; class II for pure mesangial disease, class III and IV were defined as proliferative disease, with the former affecting <50% of glomeruli and latter >50%. Class V was for membranous changes. This was modified in 1982, which include replacement of "focal proliferative" term to "focal segmental" GN and addition of a new category, class VI, which denoted advanced sclerosing GN (**Table 3**) [62].

Due to inconsistencies and ambiguities of the available classification criteria, under the auspices of International Society of Nephrology/Renal Pathology Society (ISN/RPS), a new classification of LN was proposed in 2003 [63]. While keeping the overall architecture of the 6 classes in LN, several significant changes were made and emphasis was given to standardisation of biopsy reports. Definition of class I was changed to normal glomeruli under light microscopy but with mesangial deposits under IF. There was also subdivision of class IV into diffuse segmental (IV-S) or diffuse global (IV-G), while terms active (A), chronic (C) or acute-on-chronic (A/C) lesions were also introduced.

The ISN/RPS classification for LN was revised in 2018; among the changes include elimination of the subdivisions of class IV into segmental (IV-S) or global (IV-G), replacement of previous denomination of active (A) and chronic (C) to the actual activity indices (maximum score for activity index is 24 and chronicity index is 12; **Table 4**), and preference for the term "hypercellularity" rather than "proliferation" [64]. The lack of classification for tubulointerstitial and vascular involvement in LN will be addressed and revised after the next (phase 2) international nephropathology working group evaluation and recommendations [64].

WHO 1974	ISN/RPS 2003	ISN/RPS 2018
Class I Normal glomeruli	*Class I* Minimal mesangial lupus nephritis	*Class I* Minimal mesangial lupus nephritis [d]
Class II Pure mesangial alteration	*Class II* Mesangial proliferative lupus nephritis	*Class II* Mesangial proliferative lupus nephritis [d]
Class III Focal proliferative glomerulonephritis	*Class III* Focal lupus nephritis [a, b]	*Class III* Focal lupus nephritis [d]
Class IV Diffuse proliferative glomerulonephritis	*Class IV* Diffuse segmental (IV-S) or global (IV-G) lupus nephritis [a, b]	*Class IV* Diffuse lupus nephritis [d]
Class V Membranous glomerulonephritis	*Class V* Membranous lupus nephritis [c]	*Class V* Membranous lupus nephritis [c, d]
	Class VI Advanced sclerosing lupus nephritis	*Class VI* Advanced sclerosing lupus nephritis [d]

***WHO**: *World Health Organisation;* **ISN/RPS**: *International Society of Nephrology/Renal Pathology Society;* **a**: *indicate the proportion of glomeruli with active and sclerotic lesions;* **b**: *indicate the proportion of glomeruli with fibrinoid necrosis and cellular crescents;* **c**: *may occur in combination with class III or IV;* **d**: *activity and chronicity indices (total scores of 24 for activity, 12 for chronicity).*

Table 3.
Lupus nephritis classification.

Items	Score	Comment
Activity Index		
Endocapillary hypercellularity	0 to 3+	0 to 3+ based on % involvement of glomeruli or tubulointerstitium. 0 = none, 1+ = <25%, 2+ = 25–50%, 3+ = > 50%.
Neutrophils/karyorrhexis	0 to 3+	
Fribrinoid necrosis	0 to 3+ (x2)	
Hyaline deposits	0 to 3+	
Cellular/fibrocellular crescents	0 to 3+ (x2)	Double weightage for fibrinoid necrosis and cellular/fibrocellular crescent.
Interstitial inflammation	0 to 3+	
TOTAL	24	
Chronicity Index		
Total glomerulosclerosis score	0 to 3+	0 to 3+ based on % involvement of glomeruli or tubulointerstitium. 0 = none, 1+ = <25%, 2+ = 25–50%, 3+ = > 50%.
Fibrous crescent	0 to 3+	
Tubular atrophy	0 to 3+	
Interstitial fibrosis	0 to 3+	
TOTAL	12	

Table 4.
Modified NIH activity and chronicity scoring system (ISN/RPS 2018).

5. Management

5.1 Current management strategies

Early treatment in LN has been shown to improve outcome; however, effective management remains a challenge. It requires a multidisciplinary team approach (MDT), ideally by rheumatologists, nephrologists and nephropathologists. The cornerstone of treatment entails corticosteroids, antimalarial, and steroid-sparing agents (conventional immunomodulators and/or biological therapies) tailored to individual patients based upon histological class and severity to achieve rapid resolution of inflammation, proteinuria <0.5–0.7 g/day by 12 months (or up to 24 months in baseline nephrotic range proteinuria) [47] and prevention of relapsing episodes.

5.1.1 Induction phase

While there is little agreement for class II LN, in active proliferative class III, IV and pure membranous class V (with nephrotic range proteinuria or proteinuria >1 g/day despite optimal use of renin-angiotensin-aldosterone system (RAAS) blockers), the current recommendation for initial induction treatment options include either low-dose intravenous cyclophosphamide (CYCi; 500 mg fortnightly infusions for 3 months) or mycophenolate mofetil (MMF; 2-3 g/day or mycophenolic acid (MPA) at equivalent dose) [47, 65–68]. This is combined with high-dose pulsed intravenous methylprednisolone followed by oral corticosteroid taper. High-dose CYCi is reserved for patients with severe LN due to its' various unfavourable side effects (mainly severe cytopenias and infection, cystitis, ovarian failure, cervical dysplasia and malignancy).

The use of calcineurin inhibitors (CNIs) namely tacrolimus (TAC) and cyclosporin (Cys) either as monotherapy or as part of a multitarget regimen therapy (with MMF/MPA and glucocorticoid) may have a favourable efficacy to induce remission. Meta-analysis in 2017 which included 45 induction trials of diverse participant background confirmed superior efficacy in induction by multitarget therapy compared to CYCi [69]; however, safety concern with its long term use mainly of chronic progressive irreversible nephrotoxicity remains an issue [70].

5.1.2 Maintenance phase

In the maintenance phase of treatment where less intensive therapy is required, MMF (1-2 g/day or MPA at equivalent dose) or azathioprine (AZA) are the drugs of choice [47, 71, 72] (with or without low dose <7.5 mg/day corticosteroid), depending on the induction regimen and plan for pregnancy. Hydroxychloroquine (HCQ) is recommended for all LN patients in the absence of contraindications [47]. Due to possible ocular toxicity, the dose should not exceed 5 mg/kg body weight and should be adjusted in patients with renal and liver disease, with regular ophthalmological screening.

5.1.3 Refractory lupus nephritis

Rituximab (RTX), although off-label, is not only indicated in patients refractory to conventional therapy or after great cumulative dose of CYCi, but also in patients of child bearing age [47, 73, 74]. Another B-cell targeting therapy which inhibits BlyS, Belimumab has recently been proven to be beneficial as add-on to the standard of care (SOC) therapy (mainly in the MMF subgroup) with primary efficacy renal response seen by week 24 and sustained through week 104 [75].

It is recommended not to discontinue immunosuppression too early as most renal flares occurs during this period. Treatment withrawal can be considered in patients with sustained complete remission for 3–5 years, with treatment deescalation prior to complete withrawal of therapy [47]. Close monitoring of patients and management of co-morbidities including blood pressure (BP) control, treatment of hyperlipidaemia with statins and proteinuria with RAAS blockers are important, while vaccination against influenza and *Streptococcus pneumoniae* are strongly recommended. Repeat renal biopsy may be considered to guide the duration of maintenance immunotherapy and may be required in patients with incomplete response or recurrent LN flares [47, 65].

5.2 Future novel therapeutic options

Developing more effective treatment strategies in LN remains a priority among clinicians and researchers across the globe; however, major challenges exist in its advancement due to the complex pathophysiology and heterogeneity, which directly impact on clinical trial design and overall outcome. Moreover, most trials are conducted with background therapy, which is difficult to control during the study and its subsequent analysis, as there is no clear definition in the SOC [76]. Notwithstanding this, extensive therapeutic strategies have emerged with wide array of novel treatments to improve patient outcomes. Major trend in current treatment landscape for LN focuses on reduction of steroid use.

There is gathering evidence, especially in more recent times, documenting the successful safe use of Belimumab, a monoclonal antibody (mAb) directed against BlyS as an add-on therapy in LN, especially in patients with low complement levels and high anti-DNA antibodies [75, 77]. It is the first targeted therapy and currently the only biological agent approved specifically for LN. There is also increasing interest in the sequential use of two B-cell targeting agents, RTX and Belimumab in active LN [78, 79] with a phase III trial already underway [80]. The rationale for this approach is due to the hypothesis that their co-administration may enhance depletion of circulating and tissue-resident autoreactive B cells.

Another potent BAFF-inhibitor, Blisibimod, was associated with reduction in steroid use, decreased proteinuria and biomarker responses in a multinational phase III trial [81]. Tabalumab, a selective mAb that neutralises both membrane and soluble BAFF, despite having the same therapeutic class, on the contrary did not yield the expected positive statistical significance results in two phase III studies involving SLE patients; however, only approximately 10% of patients in these studies had renal involvement [82, 83].

Voclosporin, a novel next generation CNIs (an analogue of cyclosporin) with enhanced calcineurin inhibition, better safety profile and consistent predictable dose response, despite initial safety concerns in the prior phase II study [84], has recently been demonstrated in a phase III trial to be highly effective for treatment of LN when combined with MMF, with acceptable safety profile, at least for the short term (52 weeks) [85]. More importantly, it has just received the approval by the United States' Food and Drug Administration (FDA) on the 22nd of January 2021, making it the only second targeted therapy approved specifically for LN [86].

There is emerging theoretical evidence for targeting autoantibody-secreting long-lived plasma cells (PCs) that recide in dedicated survival niches in the bone marrow or inflammed tissues of LN patients. Bortezomib, a proteasome inhibitor has been shown to be effective in both animal models and real-world setting but is limited by treatment related toxicity [87–89]. Recently, Ostendorf and colleagues have demosntrated succesful use of Daratumumab, a mAb that targets CD38 and depletes PCs with acceptable safety profile in a patient with refractory LN [90]. The experience of its use however is still limited and more data will be required.

Obinutuzumab, a novel anti-CD20 mAb demonstrated encouraging sustained 18-months B-cell depletion and renal response in a phase II trial with further evaluation in phase III trial underway (can be accessed at ClinicalTrials.gov with identification number: NCT04221477) [91]. BI 655064 (anti CD40 mAb; NCT02770170) has recently completed a phase II trial as add-on therapy to SOC treatment in active LN and awaiting evaluation. Other biological agents currently undergoing clinical trials in the treatment of LN include Anifrolumab (Type I IFN receptor mAb; NCT02547922) in phase II, while Dapirolizumab (pegylated anti CD40 ligand; NCT04294667) and Secukinumab (anti-IL-17 mAb; NCT04181762) are both in phase III trials [92].

A pipeline of novel agents in LN are being developed or asssesed in clinical trials including Ravulizumab (novel anti complement C5 antibody; NCT04564339), Guselkumab (IL-23 inhibitor; NCT04376827), Itolizumab, (anti CD6 antibody; NCT04128579), KZR-616 (proteasome inhibitor; NCT03393013), Iguratimod (novel small molecule; NCT02936375), and BMS-986165 (novel tyrosine kinase 2 (TYK2) inhibitor; NCT03943147) among many others [92].

Targeting the JAK/STAT signalling pathway with Tofacitinib, or CP-690, 550 have been shown to be effective in murine LN model and may potentially serve as therapeutic target in LN [93, 94]. Successful Bruton's Tyrosine Kinase (BTK) inhibition in several studies involving mice LN models supports *Kong et al.* finding of significantly upregulated BTK expression in glomerulus of LN patients and may potentially be a therapeutic target in LN [95–97].

Despite looking promising in SLE, a placebo-controlled phase II/III study to evaluate Atacicept (recombinant fusion protein that inhibits BAFF/BLyS or APRIL) in combination with MMF and corticosteroids in active LN patients was prematurely terminated due to unexpected substantial decline in serum IgG and serious pneumonia infections in Atacicept-treated patients [98, 99]. Abatacept, a recombinant fusion protein co-stimulation modulator, trialled as add on to SOC in LN failed the primary end point of a phase III trial despite demonstarating more rapid reduction of proteinuria and earlier sustained remission [100].

Newer treatment paradigms showing promising results include succesful use of autologous haematopoietic and allogeneic mesenchymal stem cell transplantations for LN in animal studies and among Asian patients [101–106] while *Yu et al.* demonstrated in vitro the protective role by vitamin D in podocyte injury induced by autoantibodies from patients with LN and suggested possible role of vitamin D as a novel therapy target in LN [107].

6. Special considerations

6.1 Pregnancy and lupus nephritis

6.1.1 Pre-pregnancy

Women of childbearing age with LN should understand and be counselled about the potential risks of pregnancy, even if she is in complete remission. Age, previous pregnancy complication, duration from last LN relapse, medication exposure, treatment adherence, blood pressure (BP) control and current disease status are among the important factors that may determine the outcome of future pregnancy. Baseline complement levels, antibody status for dsDNA, SS-A and SS-B, presence of antiphospholipid antibodies (aPL; notably lupus anticoagulant antibody) and urinalysis for proteinuria should be obtained prior to pregnancy.

Possible maternal complications include flare of nephritis, uncontrolled hypertension, pre-eclampsia, risk of Caesarean section, worsening renal function and thrombosis. Foetal risks include prematurity, growth retardation, congenital heart block and intrauterine death [108]. Patients with active disease at conception, uncontrolled hypertension, proteinuria of >1 g/day and abnormal renal function have the highest risk for complications; therefore, good control of disease prior to pregnancy is critically important to optimise pregnancy outcome and ideally the pregnancy should be planned.

Patients on MMF should be transitioned to pregnancy-safe immunosuppressive drugs such as AZA or TAC, while HCQ should be continued throughout pregnancy. MMF exposure especially after the first trimester increases the risk of miscarriage and congenital malformation [109], and practically should be stopped at least 3–6 months prior to conception to ensure disease control is maintained with the new agent(s) [47]. CYC is also teratogenic, associated with premature ovarian failure and increases miscarriage rate [110].

RAAS blockers should ideally be stopped before conception due to possible teratogenicity risk [111]; however, later publications seemed to suggest that they may be safe to be used until pregnancy is confirmed [112]. This is important especially for those who have residual proteinuria as attempt to conceive may take months or even years of effort. Stopping RAAS blockers early on in these patients would essentially exclude them from its' benefits.

6.1.2 During pregnancy

Multidisciplinary team approach is important during pregnancy and should ideally involve the obstetrician, neonatologist, nephrologist and rheumatologist. Majority of patients (80%) with quiescent LN would have successful pregnancies [113]; however, about a third may relapse during pregnancy [108]. Identification of patients who are at higher risk is important when pregnancy begins, as these patients will require closer observation to ensure good maternal and foetal outcomes (**Table 5**) [109, 114–118].

Baseline risk assessment	Possible complication
Active disease during conception	Pregnancy loss, pre-eclampsia, IUGR, prematurity [114]
Proteinuria >1 g/day	Worsening renal function, pre-eclampsia [115]
Uncontrolled hypertension	Pregnancy loss, IUGR, prematurity, pre-eclampsia [114]
Presence of SS-A antibody	Neonatal lupus (congenital heart block) [116]
History of recent acute kidney injury	Pre-eclampsia, IUGR and prematurity [117]
Chronic kidney disease	Worsening renal function, prematurity, IUGR, preeclampsia [118]
Mycophenolate exposure during pregnancy	Miscarriage and embryopathy involving ear, mouth, finger and ocular malformation [109]

**IUGR: Intra-uterine growth retardation.*

Table 5.
Baseline risk assessment during pregnancy.

During early pregnancy, BP would usually remain normal even in patients who required antihypertensive before pregnancy. Gradually, BP may rise as pregnancy progresses, requiring reintroduction of hypertensive medications such as labetalol, methyldopa or nifedipine. BP control should be targeted to be less than 140/90 mmHg [119]. As these patients are at higher risk to develop pre-eclampsia, high dose calcium supplementation and aspirin should be prescribed before entering 16 weeks of gestation [120, 121]. Ultrasound screening including uterine and umbilical artery Doppler to detect early signs of placental insufficiency may be performed at regular interval, especially in high-risk patients.

Hydroxychloroquine is safe during pregnancy and discontinuation has been associated with lupus flare. It also significantly reduces the risk of foetal congenital heart block in patients with positive SS-A (anti-Ro) [116]. Other drugs for consideration in LN and compatible with pregnancy include AZA, CNIs (TAC, Cys), plasma exchange and intravenous immunoglobulins. Data on RTX in pregnancy is limited, although some clinicians have used it safely in early trimester without apparent complication [122]. LN flare during pregnancy can be treated with drugs mentioned above and with addition or increased dosage of steroid. Pulsed intravenous methylprednisolone may be given during severe flares, followed by oral prednisolone [114]. While use of steroid is associated with elevated BP and new onset diabetes, it is probably not related to cleft lip and palate as previously thought [123, 124] (**Table 6**).

Medication	Pregnancy	Breastfeeding
Cyclophosphamide	Increased risk of teratogenicity, especially in 1st trimester	May cause infants' bone marrow suppression
Mycophenolate	Increased risk of congenital malformation and miscarriage	Limited data, not recommended
Azathioprine	Relatively safe. Alternative to mycophenolate	Relatively safe
Hydroxychloroquine	Relatively safe. Improve outcome in antiphospholipid syndrome	Relatively safe
Glucocorticoids	Increase risk of hypertension, preeclampsia, GDM. May have neutral effect on cleft lip and palate	Relatively safe
Calcineurin inhibitor	Increase risk of high blood pressure and diabetes. Relatively safe	Relatively safe
Rituximab	Limited data. No teratogenic effect in animal. 1st trimester use may be possible.	Limited data
Immunoglobulin	Safe in pregnancy. Headache & rash common side effect	Relatively safe

**GDM: Gestational diabetes mellitus.*

Table 6.
Summary of immunosuppressive drugs during perinatal period.

Differentiating between pre-eclampsia and LN flare in pregnancy may be difficult, especially after 20 weeks gestation. Features like proteinuria, high BP, thrombocytopenia and renal impairment are common in both conditions. Red cell cast in urine, abnormal level of complements and anti-dsDNA may point toward LN flare [125]. Elevated soluble fms-like tyrosine kinase 1 (sFlt1)/placental growth factor (PlGF) ratio may assist in predicting pre-eclampsia [126, 127] although not commonly available in clinical practice.

Renal biopsy may be required during pregnancy but poses increased risk of complications. In a systematic review involving data on renal biopsies performed during pregnancy, overall complication rate was higher at 7%, compared to 1% when performed post-partum. Importantly, 4 biopsies during pregnancy had major bleeding complications that required blood transfusion, with median gestational age of 25 weeks; hence, biopsy should only be considered early during the course of pregnancy when results may lead to changes in therapy. Biopsy should be considered if LN flare is suspected and to distinguish it from pre-eclampsia, with finding of glomerular endotheliosis would suggest the latter [128].

Multidisciplinary team approach and patients' engagement are prudent during severe LN flare, as pregnancy termination may be considered with risks and benefits weighed carefully, so that patient can be treated with urgent cytotoxic drugs. Overall rate for preterm delivery and Caesarean section are higher in patients with LN. For patients with non-active disease, delivery at term should be aimed. In those likely to deliver prematurely, dexamethasone should be given to accelerate foetal lung maturation. Delivery should be aimed after 34 weeks to minimise neonatal adverse outcomes; nonetheless, this strategy relies on the overall clinical picture. Timing of delivery is determined by usual obstetric indications and risk of renal deterioration. Mode of delivery does not seem to affect maternal renal function and again should be based on the usual indications accordingly [129].

6.1.3 *After pregnancy*

The WHO recommends breastfeeding for all babies until 6 months of age, even in patients on immunosuppressive therapy. Although studies found trace amount of immunosuppressives excreted into breast milk, the amount absorbed by infant is negligible and do not exert any clinical effect [130]. Hence, immunosuppressives deemed safe during pregnancy such as corticosteroid, AZA and CNIs can be safely taken during breastfeeding [114]. Post-partum, regular antihypertensive drugs such as amlodipine or bisoprolol can be reinstated and RAAS blockers such as enalapril or captopril can be safely used during breastfeeding [131] (**Table 6**).

Postpartum risk of thromboembolic disease increases in SLE especially in active LN patients with nephrotic-range proteinuria. Preventative measure with heparin during postpartum period is controversial, but may be considered in active LN patients with risk factors such as advanced age, obesity, Caesarean section delivery, and pre-eclampsia [132]. For patients with chronic kidney disease and significant proteinuria during pregnancy, careful monitoring after delivery is required as decline in renal function may accelerate within 6–12 months postpartum, despite having stable renal function during pregnancy [133].

6.2 Renal transplantation in lupus nephritis

Approximately 10–20% of patients with LN will progress to ESRD, with young female of African ancestry having the highest risk [8, 134]. In general, outcome for renal transplant is better compared to dialysis particularly with preemptive transplantation, including in patients with LN [135]. However, many patients may not be in complete remission despite dialysis initiation, making preemptive transplantation difficult. Current guidelines suggest that clinical lupus activity and ideally, serologically should be quiescent for 6 months and on no or minimal immunosuppression prior to transplantation [47, 136]. Even if on dialysis, the waiting time for transplant should be maximally shortened to reduce potential risk of graft failure [137].

Although the benefit of transplantation is clear, earlier studies have suggested that LN patients may have worse survival outcome compared to ESRD patients of other aetiologies; however, more contemporary studies seem to abrogate this finding [138]. Clinically relevant recurrence rate of SLE post transplantation is less than 5%, but it increases the risk of graft failure [136]. The rate may even be higher if electron microscopy finding is included and protocol biopsy implemented; nevertheless, the lower rate is probably due to the similar immunosuppressive therapy used in both transplant recipient and active LN.

During pre-transplant evaluation, particular attention should be given to screening of aPL as its' presence increases the risk of graft thrombosis. Patients with APS would require careful consideration of perioperative anticoagulation to prevent graft loss. Presence of anti-dsDNA or low complement level is not a predictor for renal transplant outcomes. SLE patients have higher risk for cardiovascular mortality hence will require careful cardiac evaluation prior to transplantation [138]. Recurrence of LN after transplantation can be treated by increasing the dose of the immunosuppressive drugs already being used post transplant. CYC may be considered in severe or aggressive disease while RTX has been used in resistant cases [139].

There is concern in LN patients of having higher risk to develop cancer with prolonged exposure to immunosuppression. Previous exposure to CYC doubles the risk for cancer post transplantation, primarily of the skin [140]. Prior use of immunosuppressive therapies before transplant also increases the risk for non-Hodgkin's lymphoma, anogenital, breast, renal and bladder cancers [141, 142]. Furthermore, prolonged corticosteroid exposure in transplanted SLE patients should adhere to the screening and treatment recommendations on bone health [143].

7. Conclusion

Emerging insights into the heterogenous immunopathogenesis of LN have lead to novel, tailored therapeutic options, resulting in significantly better disease control and prolonged remission among patients; nonetheless, more in-depth studies are required to better understand the pathogenesis while novel therapies continue to be tested. The advent of signature biomarkers show promise in diagnosis, evaluation and management of LN and will continue to be validated for meaningful real-world application. Timely diagnosis, prompt treat-to-target treatment, MDT approach and adherence to therapy are important factors to preserve renal function, prevent disease progression and significantly improve patients' overall outcome.

Better understanding of disease pathways and discoveries with subsequent validation of biomarkers will provide opportunity for improvement in early detection, prognostic and disease severity prediction, subgroups stratification, treatment adherence assessment, and decision for best treatment option in a timely manner. Studies targeting a single organ or specific subgroup with similar disease severity, duration and background SOC therapy will assist in better assesment of drug effectiveness and accelerate drug development in LN.

Author details

Fahd Adeeb[1*] and Wan Ahmad Hafiz Wan Md Adnan[2]

1 Department of Rheumatology, University Hospital Kerry, Kerry, Ireland

2 Department of Nephrology, University Malaya, Kuala Lumpur, Malaysia

*Address all correspondence to: fahd_adeeb@yahoo.com

References

[1] Anders H, Saxena R, Zhao M, Parodis I, Salmon JE, Mohan *C. lupus* nephritis. Nat Rev Dis Primers 2020; 6: 7

[2] Mohan, C., Putterman, C. Genetics and pathogenesis of systemic lupus erythematosus and lupus nephritis. Nat Rev Nephrol 2015; 11: 329-341

[3] Gonzalez-Crespo MR, Lopez-Fernandez JI, Usera G, Poveda MJ, Gomez-Reino JJ. Outcome of silent lupus nephritis. Semin Arthritis Rheum 1996; 26: 468-76

[4] Wakasugi D, Gono T, Kawaguchi Y, Hara M, Koseki Y, Katsumata Y, et al. Frequency of Class III and IV Nephritis in Systemic Lupus Erythematosus without Clinical Renal Involvement: An Analysis of Predictive Measures. J Rheumatol 2012; 39: 79-85

[5] Jorge A, Wallace ZS, Zhang Y, Lu N, Costenbader KH, Choi HK. All-Cause and Cause-Specific Mortality Trends of End-Stage Renal Disease Due to Lupus Nephritis From 1995 to 2014. Arthritis Rheumatol 2019; 71: 403-410

[6] Tektonidou MG, Dasgupta A, Ward MM. Risk of End-Stage Renal Disease in Patients With Lupus Nephritis, 1971-2015: A Systematic Review and Bayesian Meta-Analysis. Arthritis Rheumatol 2016; 68: 1432-41

[7] Davidson A. What is damaging the kidney in lupus nephritis? *Nat Rev Rheumatol* 2016; 12: 143-153

[8] Maroz N, Segal M*S. lupus* nephritis and end-stage kidney disease. Am J Med Sci 2013; 346: 319-23

[9] Rees F, Doherty M, Grainge M, Davenport G, Lanyon P, Zhang W. The incidence and prevalence of systemic lupus erythematosus in the UK, 1999-2012. Annals of the rheumatic diseases 2016; 75: 136-41

[10] Rees F, Doherty M, Grainge MJ, Lanyon P, Zhang W. The worldwide incidence and prevalence of systemic lupus erythematosus: a systematic review of epidemiological studies. Rheumatology 2017; 56: 1945-61

[11] Stojan G, Petri M. Epidemiology of systemic lupus erythematosus: an update. Curr Opin Rheumatol 2018; 30: 144-50

[12] Dall'Era M, Cisternas MG, Snipes K, Herrinton LJ, Gordon C, Helmick CG. The Incidence and Prevalence of Systemic Lupus Erythematosus in San Francisco County, California: The California Lupus Surveillance Project. Arthritis Rheumatol 2017; 69: 1996-2005

[13] Yeh KW, Yu CH, Chan PC, Horng JT, Huang JL. Burden of systemic lupus erythematosus in Taiwan: a population-based survey. Rheumatol Int 2013; 33: 1805-11

[14] Jakes RW, Bae SC, Louthrenoo W, Mok CC, Navarra SV, Kwon N. Systematic review of the epidemiology of systemic lupus erythematosus in the Asia-Pacific region: prevalence, incidence, clinical features, and mortality. Arthritis Care Res 2012; 64: 159-68

[15] Imran TF, Yick F, Verma S, Estiverne C, Ogbonnaya-Odor C, Thiruvarudsothy S, et al. Lupus nephritis: an update. Clin Exp Nephrol 2016; 20: 1-13

[16] Bastian HM, Roseman JM, McGwin G, Jr., Alarcón GS, Friedman AW, Fessler BJ, et al. Systemic lupus erythematosus in three ethnic groups. XII. Risk factors for lupus nephritis after Diagnosis*. lupus* 2002; 11: 152-60

[17] Boodhoo KD, Liu S, Zuo X. Impact of sex disparities on the clinical

manifestations in patients with systemic lupus erythematosus: A systematic review and meta-analysis. Medicine 2016; 95: e4272

[18] Yap DY, Tang CS, Ma MK, Lam MF, Chan TM. Survival analysis and causes of mortality in patients with lupus nephritis. Nephrol Dial Transplant 2012; 27: 3248-54

[19] Wardowska A, Komorniczak M, Bułło-Piontecka B, Dębska-Ślizień MA, Pikuła M. Transcriptomic and Epigenetic Alterations in Dendritic Cells Correspond With Chronic Kidney Disease in Lupus Nephritis. Front Immunol 2019;10: 2026

[20] Zhao M, Zhou Y, Zhu B, Wan M, Jiang T, Tan Q, Liu Y, Jiang J, Luo S, Tan Y, et al. IFI44L promoter methylation as a blood biomarker for systemic lupus erythematosus. Ann Rheum 2016; 75: 1998-2006

[21] Yung S, Chan TM. Autoantibodies and resident renal cells in the pathogenesis of lupus nephritis: getting to know the unknown. Clin Dev Immunol 2012; 2012: 139365

[22] Devarapu SK, Anders HJ. Toll-like receptors in lupus nephritis. J Biomed Sci 2018; 25: 35

[23] Santiago-Raber ML, Baudino L, Izui S. Emerging roles of TLR7 and TLR9 in murine SLE. J Autoimmun. 2009; 33: 231-8

[24] Bergtold A, Gavhane A, D'Agati V, Madaio M, Clynes R. FcR-bearing myeloid cells are responsible for triggering murine lupus nephritis. J Immunol 2006; 177: 7287-95

[25] Werwitzke S, Trick D, Sondermann P, Kamino K, Schlegelberger B, Kniesch K, Tiede A, Jacob U, Schmidt RE, Witte T. Treatment of lupus-prone NZB/NZW F1 mice with recombinant soluble Fc gamma receptor II (CD32). Ann Rheum Dis 2008; 67: 154-61

[26] Pickering MC, Botto M. Are anti-C1q antibodies different from other SLE autoantibodies? Nat Rev Rheumatol. 2010; 6: 490-3.

[27] Stojan G, Petri M. Anti-C1q in systemic lupus Erythematosus. *lupus* 2016; 25: 873-877

[28] Rönnblom L, Leonard D. Interferon pathway in SLE: one key to unlocking the mystery of the disease. Lupus Sci Med. 2019; 6: e000270

[29] Chalmers SA, Garcia SJ, Reynolds JA, Herlitz L, Putterman C. NF-kB signalling in myeloid cells mediates the pathogenesis of immune-mediated nephritis. J Autoimmun 2019; 98: 33-43

[30] Hiepe F, Radbruch A. Plasma cells as an innovative target in autoimmune disease with renal manifestations. Nat Rev Nephrol 2016; 12: 232-40

[31] Kang S, Fedoriw Y, Brenneman EK, Truong YK, Kikly K, Vilen BJ. BAFF induces tertiary lymphoid structures and positions T cells within the glomeruli during lupus nephritis. J Immunol 2017; 198: 2602-11

[32] Koga T, Ichinose K, Tsokos GC. T cells and IL-17 in lupus nephritis. Clin Immunol 2017;185:95-99

[33] Martinez J, Cunha LD, Park S, Yang M, Lu Q, Orchard R, et al. Noncanonical autophagy inhibits the autoinflammatory, lupus-like response to dying cells. Nature 2016; 533: 115-119

[34] Qi YY, Zhou XJ, Cheng FJ, Hou P, Ren YL, Wang S, et al. Increased autophagy is cytoprotective against podocyte injury induced by antibody and interferon-alpha in lupus nephritis. Ann Rheum Dis 2018; 77: 1799-1809

[35] Zhou XJ, Klionsky DJ, Zhang H. Podocytes and autophagy: a potential therapeutic target in lupus nephritis. Autophagy 2019; 15: 908-912

[36] Ko K, Wang J, Perper S, et al. Bcl-2 as a Therapeutic Target in Human Tubulointerstitial Inflammation. Arthritis Rheumatol 2016; 68: 2740-2751

[37] Tanha N, Troelsen L, From Hermansen ML, Kjær L, Faurschou M, Garred P, Jacobsen S. MBL2 gene variants coding for mannose-binding lectin deficiency are associated with increased risk of nephritis in Danish patients with systemic lupus Erythematosus. *lupus* 2014; 23: 1105-11

[38] Wu S, Wang J, Li F. Dysregulation of PTEN caused by the underexpression of microRNA-130b is associated with the severity of lupus nephritis. Mol Med Rep 2018; 17: 7966-7972

[39] Pieterse E, van der Vlag J. Breaking immunological tolerance in systemic lupus erythematosus. Front Immunol 2014; 5: 164

[40] Gupta S, Kaplan MJ. The role of neutrophils and NETosis in autoimmune and renal diseases. Nat Rev Nephrol 2016; 12: 402-413

[41] Yu F, Haas M, Glassock R, Zhao MH. Redefining lupus nephritis: clinical implications of pathophysiologic subtypes. Nat Rev Nephrol 2017;13: 483-495

[42] Celhar T, Lu HK, Benso L, Rakhilina L, Lee HY, Tripathi S, et al. TLR7 Protein Expression in Mild and Severe Lupus-Prone Models Is Regulated in a Leukocyte, Genetic, and IRAK4 Dependent Manner. Front Immunol 2019; 10: 1546

[43] Dillon SP, Kurien BT, Li S, Bruner GR, Kaufman KM, Harley JB, Gaffney PM, Wallace DJ, Weisman MH, Scofield RH. Sex chromosome aneuploidies among men with systemic lupus erythematosus. J Autoimmun 2012; 38: J129-34

[44] Souyris M, Cenac C, Azar P, Daviaud D, Canivet A, Grunenwald S, et al. TLR7 escapes X chromosome inactivation in immune cells. Sci Immunol 2018; 3: eaap8855

[45] Soliman S, Mohan *C. lupus* nephritis biomarkers. Clin Immunol 2017; 185: 10-20

[46] Mavragani CP, Fragoulis GE, Somarakis G, Drosos A, Tzioufas AG, Moutsopoulos HM. Clinical and laboratory predictors of distinct histopathogical features of lupus nephritis. Medicine 2015; 94: e829

[47] Fanouriakis A, Kostopoulou M, Cheema K, Anders HJ, Aringer M, Bajema I, et al. 2019 Update of the Joint European League Against Rheumatism and European Renal Association-European Dialysis and Transplant Association (EULAR/ERA-EDTA) recommendations for the management of lupus nephritis. Ann Rheum Dis 2020; 79: 713-23

[48] Hogan JJ, Mocanu M, Berns JS. The Native Kidney Biopsy: Update and Evidence for Best Practice. Clin J Am Soc Nephrol 2016; 11: 354-62

[49] Corapi KM, Chen JL, Balk EM, Gordon CE. Bleeding complications of native kidney biopsy: a systematic review and meta-analysis. Am J Kidney Dis 2012; 60: 62-73

[50] Korbet SM, Volpini KC, Whittier WL. Percutaneous renal biopsy of native kidneys: a single-center experience of 1,055 biopsies. Am J Nephrol 2014; 39: 153-62

[51] Marwah DS, Korbet SM. Timing of complications in percutaneous renal biopsy: what is the optimal period of

observation? Am J Kidney Dis 1996; 28: 47-52

[52] Schorr M, Roshanov PS, Weir MA, House AA. Frequency, Timing, and Prediction of Major Bleeding Complications From Percutaneous Renal Biopsy. Can J Kidney Health Dis 2020; 7: 2054358120923527

[53] Waldo B, Korbet SM, Freimanis MG, Lewis EJ. The value of post-biopsy ultrasound in predicting complications after percutaneous renal biopsy of native kidneys. Nephrol Dial Transplant 2009; 24: 2433-9

[54] Moroni G, Depetri F, Ponticelli C. *lupus* nephritis: When and how often to biopsy and what does it mean? J Autoimmun 2016; 74: 27-40

[55] Narváez J, Ricse M, Gomà M, Mitjavila F, Fulladosa X, Capdevila O, et al. The value of repeat biopsy in lupus nephritis flares. Medicine 2017; 96: e7099

[56] De Rosa M, Azzato F, Toblli JE, De Rosa G, Fuentes F, Nagaraja HN, et al. A prospective observational cohort study highlights kidney biopsy findings of lupus nephritis patients in remission who flare following withdrawal of maintenance therapy. Kidney Int 2018; 94: 788-94

[57] Hochberg MC. Updating the American College of Rheumatology revised criteria for the classification of systemic lupus erythematosus. Arthritis Rheum 1997; 40: 1725

[58] Petri M, Orbai AM, Alarcón GS, Gordon C, Merrill JT, Fortin PR, et al. Derivation and validation of the Systemic Lupus International Collaborating Clinics classification criteria for systemic lupus erythematosus. Arthritis Rheum 2012; 64: 2677-86

[59] Aringer M, Costenbader K, Daikh D, Brinks R, Mosca M, Ramsey-Goldman R, et al. 2019 European League Against Rheumatism/ American College of Rheumatology Classification Criteria for Systemic Lupus Erythematosus. Arthritis Rheum 2019; 71: 1400-12

[60] Ishizaki J, Saito K, Nawata M, Mizuno Y, Tokunaga M, Sawamukai N, et al. Low complements and high titre of anti-Sm antibody as predictors of histopathologically proven silent lupus nephritis without abnormal urinalysis in patients with systemic lupus erythematosus. Rheumatology 2015; 54: 405-12

[61] Kudose S, Santoriello D, Bomback AS, Stokes MB, D'Agati VD, Markowitz GS. Sensitivity and Specificity of Pathologic Findings to Diagnose Lupus Nephritis. Clin J Am Soc Nephrol 2019; 14: 1605

[62] Churg J, Sobin LH. Renal disease. Classification and Atlas of Glomerular Disease. Tokyo, Igaku-Shoin, 1982; 359

[63] Weening JJ, D'Agati VD, Schwartz MM, Seshan SV, Alpers CE, Appel GB, et al. The classification of glomerulonephritis in systemic lupus erythematosus revisited. Kidney Int 2004; 65: 521-30

[64] Bajema IM, Wilhelmus S, Alpers CE, Bruijn JA, Colvin RB, Cook HT, et al. Revision of the International Society of Nephrology/ Renal Pathology Society classification for lupus nephritis: clarification of definitions, and modified National Institutes of Health activity and chronicity indices. Kidney Int 2018; 93: 789-96

[65] Kostopoulou M, Adamichou C, Bertsias G. An Update on the Diagnosis and Management of Lupus Nephritis. Curr Rheumatol Rep 2020; 22: 30

[66] Palmer SC, Tunnicliffe DJ, Singh-Grewal D, Mavridis D, Tonelli M,

Johnson DW, et al. Induction and Maintenance Immunosuppression Treatment of Proliferative Lupus Nephritis: A Network Meta-analysis of Randomized Trials. Am J Kidney Dis 2017; 70: 324-336

[67] Houssiau FA, Vasconcelos C, D'Cruz D, Sebastiani GD, Garrido Ed Ede R, Danieli MG, et al. Immunosuppressive therapy in lupus nephritis: the Euro-Lupus Nephritis Trial, a randomized trial of low-dose versus high-dose intravenous cyclophosphamide. Arthritis Rheum 2002; 46: 2121-31

[68] Rathi M, Goyal A, Jaryal A, Sharma A, Gupta PK, Ramachandran R, et al. Comparison of low-dose intravenous cyclophosphamide with oral mycophenolate mofetil in the treatment of lupus nephritis. Kidney Int 2016; 89: 235-42

[69] Palmer SC, Tunnicliffe DJ, Singh-Grewal D, Mavridis D, Tonelli M, Johnson DW, et al. Induction and Maintenance Immunosuppression Treatment of Proliferative Lupus Nephritis: A Network Meta-analysis of Randomized Trials. Am J Kidney Dis 2017; 70: 324-336

[70] Nankivell BJ, P'Ng CH, O'Connell PJ, Chapman JR. Calcineurin Inhibitor Nephrotoxicity Through the Lens of Longitudinal Histology: Comparison of Cyclosporine and Tacrolimus Eras. Transplantation 2016; 100: 1723-31

[71] Tamirou F, D'Cruz D, Sangle S, Remy P, Vasconcelos C, Fiehn C, et al. Long-term follow-up of the MAINTAIN Nephritis Trial, comparing azathioprine and mycophenolate mofetil as maintenance therapy of lupus nephritis. Ann Rheum Dis 2016; 75: 526-31

[72] Dooley MA, Jayne D, Ginzler EM, Isenberg D, Olsen NJ, Wofsy D, et al. Mycophenolate versus azathioprine as maintenance therapy for lupus nephritis. N Engl J Med 2011; 365: 1886-95

[73] Díaz-Lagares C, Croca S, Sangle S, Vital EM, Catapano F, Martínez-Berriotxoa A, et al; UK-BIOGEAS Registry. Efficacy of rituximab in 164 patients with biopsy-proven lupus nephritis: pooled data from European cohorts. Autoimmun Rev 2012; 11: 357-64

[74] Condon MB, Ashby D, Pepper RJ, Cook HT, Levy JB, Griffith M, et al. Prospective observational single-centre cohort study to evaluate the effectiveness of treating lupus nephritis with rituximab and mycophenolate mofetil but no oral steroids. Ann Rheum Dis 2013; 72: 1280-6

[75] Furie R, Rovin BH, Houssiau F, Malvar A, Teng YKO, Contreras G, et al. Two-Year, Randomized, Controlled Trial of Belimumab in Lupus Nephritis. N Engl J Med 2020; 383: 1117-1128

[76] Dall'Era M, Bruce IN, Gordon C, Manzi S, McCaffrey J, Lipsky PE. Current challenges in the development of new treatments for lupus. Ann Rheum Dis 2019; 78: 729-735

[77] Dooley MA, Houssiau F, Aranow C, D'Cruz DP, Askanase A, Roth DA, et al; BLISS-52 and -76 Study Groups. Effect of belimumab treatment on renal outcomes: results from the phase 3 belimumab clinical trials in patients with SLE. Lupus 2013; 22: 63-72

[78] Gualtierotti R, Borghi MO, Gerosa M, Schioppo T, Larghi P, Geginat J, et al. Successful sequential therapy with rituximab and belimumab in patients with active systemic lupus erythematosus: a case series. Clin Exp Rheumatol 2018; 36: 643-647

[79] Simonetta F, Allali D, Roux-Lombard P, Chizzolini C. Successful treatment of refractory lupus

nephritis by the sequential use of rituximab and belimumab. Joint Bone Spine 2017; 84: 235-236

[80] Teng YKO, Bruce IN, Diamond B, Furie RA, van Vollenhoven RF, Gordon D, et al. Phase III, multicentre, randomised, double-blind, placebo-controlled, 104-week study of subcutaneous belimumab administered in combination with rituximab in adults with systemic lupus erythematosus (SLE): BLISS-BELIEVE study protocol. BMJ Open 2019; 9: e025687

[81] Merrill JT, Shanahan WR, Scheinberg M, Kalunian KC, Wofsy D, Martin RS. Phase III trial results with blisibimod, a selective inhibitor of B-cell activating factor, in subjects with systemic lupus erythematosus (SLE): results from a randomised, double-blind, placebo-controlled trial. Ann Rheum Dis 2018; 77: 883-889

[82] Isenberg DA, Petri M, Kalunian K, Tanaka Y, Urowitz MB, Hoffman RW, et al. Efficacy and safety of subcutaneous tabalumab in patients with systemic lupus erythematosus: results from ILLUMINATE-1, a 52-week, phase III, multicentre, randomised, double-blind, placebo-controlled study. Ann Rheum Dis 2016; 75: 323-31

[83] Merrill JT, van Vollenhoven RF, Buyon JP, Furie RA, Stohl W, Morgan-Cox M, et al. Efficacy and safety of subcutaneous tabalumab, a monoclonal antibody to B-cell activating factor, in patients with systemic lupus erythematosus: results from ILLUMINATE-2, a 52-week, phase III, multicentre, randomised, double-blind, placebo-controlled study. Ann Rheum Dis 2016; 75: 332-40

[84] Rovin BH, Solomons N, Pendergraft WF 3rd, Dooley MA, Tumlin J, Romero-Diaz J, et al; AURA-LV Study Group. A randomized, controlled double-blind study comparing the efficacy and safety of dose-ranging voclosporin with placebo in achieving remission in patients with active lupus nephritis. Kidney Int 2019; 95: 219-231

[85] Arriens C, Polyakova S, Adzerikho I, Rhandawa S, Solomons N. OP0277 AURORA Phase 3 Study Demonstrates Voclosporin Statistical Superiority Over Standard of Care in Lupus Nephritis (LN). Ann Rheum Dis 2020; 79: 172-173

[86] U.S Food and Drug Administration, Center for Drug Evaluation and Research. Lupkynis (voclosporin) approval letter. January 22, 2021. Retrieved 28/1/21 from www.accessdata.fda.gov/drugsatfda_docs/appletter/2021/213716Orig1s000ltr.pdf

[87] Neubert K, Meister S, Moser K, Weisel F, Maseda D, Amann K, et al. The proteasome inhibitor bortezomib depletes plasma cells and protects mice with lupus-like disease from nephritis. Nat Med 2008; 14: 748-55

[88] Alexander T, Sarfert R, Klotsche J, Kühl AA, Rubbert-Roth A, Lorenz HM, et al. The proteasome inhibitior bortezomib depletes plasma cells and ameliorates clinical manifestations of refractory systemic lupus erythematosus. Ann Rheum Dis 2015; 74: 1474-8

[89] Segarra A, Arredondo KV, Jaramillo J, Jatem E, Salcedo MT, Agraz I, Ramos N, Carnicer C, Valtierra N, Ostos E. Efficacy and safety of bortezomib in refractory lupus nephritis: a single-center experience. Lupus 2020; 29: 118-125

[90] Ostendorf L, Burns M, Durek P, Heinz GA, Heinrich F, Garantziotis P, Enghard P, Richter U, Biesen R, Schneider U, Knebel F, Burmester G, Radbruch A, Mei HE, Mashreghi MF, Hiepe F, Alexander T. Targeting CD38 with Daratumumab in Refractory Systemic Lupus Erythematosus. N Engl J Med 2020; 383: 1149-1155

[91] Furie R, Aroca G, Alvarez A, Fragoso-Loyo H, Zuta Santillan E, Rovin B, et al. Two-Year Results from a Randomized Controlled Study of Obinutuzumab for Proliferative Lupus Nephritis [asbtract]. Arthritis Rheumatol 2020; 72 (suppl 10)

[92] United States National Library of Medicine database for clinical trials. Can be assessed at ClinicalTrials.gov with subsequent insertion of identification number

[93] Zhou M, Guo C, Li X, Huang Y, Li M, Zhang T, et al. JAK/STAT signalling controls the fate of $CD8^{+}CD103^{+}$tissue-resident memory T cell in lupus nephritis. J Autoimmun 2020; 109: 102424

[94] Ripoll È, de Ramon L, Draibe Bordignon J, Merino A, Bolaños N, Goma M, et al. JAK3-STAT pathway blocking benefits in experimental lupus nephritis. Arthritis Res Ther 2016; 18: 134. Erratum in: Arthritis Res Ther 2016; 18: 152

[95] Kim YY, Park KT, Jang SY, Lee KH, Byun JY, Suh KH, et al. HM71224, a selective Bruton's tyrosine kinase inhibitor, attenuates the development of murine lupus. Arthritis Res Ther 2017; 19: 211

[96] Chalmers SA, Glynn E, Garcia SJ, Panzenbeck M, Pelletier J, Dimock J, et al. BTK inhibition ameliorates kidney disease in spontaneous lupus nephritis. Clin Immunol 2018; 197: 205-218

[97] Kong W, Deng W, Sun Y, Huang S, Zhang Z, Shi B, et al. Increased expression of Bruton's tyrosine kinase in peripheral blood is associated with lupus nephritis. Clin Rheumatol 2018; 37: 43-49

[98] Merrill JT, Wallace DJ, Wax S, Kao A, Fraser PA, Chang P, et al; ADDRESS II Investigators. Efficacy and Safety of Atacicept in Patients With Systemic Lupus Erythematosus: Results of a Twenty-Four-Week, Multicenter, Randomized, Double-Blind, Placebo-Controlled, Parallel-Arm, Phase IIb Study. Arthritis Rheumatol 2018; 70: 266-276. Erratum in: Arthritis Rheumatol 2018; 70: 467

[99] Ginzler EM, Wax S, Rajeswaran A, Copt S, Hillson J, Ramos E, et al. Atacicept in combination with MMF and corticosteroids in lupus nephritis: results of a prematurely terminated trial. Arthritis Res Ther 2012; 14: R33

[100] Furie R, Dooley M, Wofsy D, Takeuchi T, Malvar A, Doria A, et al. OP0253 A phase III randomised, double-blind, placebo-controlled study to evaluate the efficacy and safety of abatacept or placebo on standard of care in patients with active class iii or iv lupus nephritis. Ann Rheum Dis 2018; 77: 176-177

[101] Bukulmez H, Horkayne-Szakaly I, Bilgin A, Baker TP, Caplan AI, Jones OY. Intrarenal injection of mesenchymal stem cell for treatment of lupus nephritis in mice - a pilot study. Lupus 2020: 961203320968897

[102] Tang X, Li W, Wen X, Zhang Z, Chen W, Yao G, et al. Transplantation of dental tissue-derived mesenchymal stem cells ameliorates nephritis in lupus mice. Ann Transl Med 2019; 7: 132

[103] Huang X, Chen W, Ren G, Zhao L, Guo J, Gong D, et al. Autologous Hematopoietic Stem Cell Transplantation for Refractory Lupus Nephritis. Clin J Am Soc Nephrol 2019; 14: 719-727

[104] Yuan X, Qin X, Wang D, Zhang Z, Tang X, Gao X, et al. Mesenchymal stem cell therapy induces FLT3L and $CD1c^{+}$ dendritic cells in systemic lupus erythematosus patients. Nat Commun 2019; 10: 2498

[105] Gu F, Wang D, Zhang H, Feng X, Gilkeson GS, Shi S, et al. Allogeneic

mesenchymal stem cell transplantation for lupus nephritis patients refractory to conventional therapy. Clin Rheumatol 2014; 33: 1611-9

[106] Leng XM, Jiang Y, Zhou DB, Tian XP, Li TS, Wang SJ, et al. Good outcome of severe lupus patients with high-dose immunosuppressive therapy and autologous peripheral blood stem cell transplantation: a 10-year follow-up study. Clin Exp Rheumatol 2017; 35: 494-499

[107] Yu Q, Qiao Y, Liu D, Liu F, Gao C, Duan J, et al. Vitamin D protects podocytes from autoantibodies induced injury in lupus nephritis by reducing aberrant autophagy. Arthritis Res Ther 2019; 21: 19

[108] Smyth A, Oliveira GH, Lahr BD, Bailey KR, Norby SM, Garovic VD. A systematic review and meta-analysis of pregnancy outcomes in patients with systemic lupus erythematosus and lupus nephritis. Clin J Am Soc Nephrol 2010; 5: 2060-8

[109] Perez-Aytes A, Marin-Reina P, Boso V, Ledo A, Carey JC, Vento M. Mycophenolate mofetil embryopathy: A newly recognized teratogenic syndrome. Eur J Med Genet 2017; 60: 16-21

[110] Rengasamy P. Congenital Malformations Attributed to Prenatal Exposure to Cyclophosphamide. Anticancer Agents Med Chem 2017; 17: 1211-1227

[111] Cooper WO, Hernandez-Diaz S, Arbogast PG, Dudley JA, Dyer S, Gideon PS, et al. Major congenital malformations after first-trimester exposure to ACE inhibitors. N Engl J Med 2006; 354: 2443-51

[112] Porta M, Hainer JW, Jansson SO, Malm A, Bilous R, Chaturvedi N, et al. Exposure to candesartan during the first trimester of pregnancy in type 1 diabetes: experience from the placebo-controlled DIabetic REtinopathy Candesartan Trials. Diabetologia 2011; 54: 1298-303

[113] Buyon JP, Kim MY, Guerra MM, Laskin CA, Petri M, Lockshin MD, et al. Predictors of Pregnancy Outcomes in Patients With Lupus: A Cohort Study. Ann Intern Med 2015; 163: 153-63

[114] Andreoli L, Bertsias GK, Agmon-Levin N, Brown S, Cervera R, Costedoat-Chalumeau N, et al. EULAR recommendations for women's health and the management of family planning, assisted reproduction, pregnancy and menopause in patients with systemic lupus erythematosus and/or antiphospholipid syndrome. Ann Rheum Dis 2017; 76: 476-85

[115] Imbasciati E, Gregorini G, Cabiddu G, Gammaro L, Ambroso G, Del Giudice A, et al. Pregnancy in CKD stages 3 to 5: fetal and maternal outcomes. Am J Kidney Dis 2007; 49: 753-62

[116] Izmirly PM, Costedoat-Chalumeau N, Pisoni CN, Khamashta MA, Kim MY, Saxena A, et al. Maternal use of hydroxychloroquine is associated with a reduced risk of recurrent anti-SSA/Ro-antibody-associated cardiac manifestations of neonatal lupus. Circulation 2012; 126: 76-82

[117] Tangren JS, Wan Md Adnan WAH, Powe CE, Ecker J, Bramham K, Hladunewich MA, et al. Risk of Preeclampsia and Pregnancy Complications in Women With a History of Acute Kidney Injury. Hypertension 2018; 72: 451-9

[118] Piccoli GB, Cabiddu G, Attini R, Vigotti FN, Maxia S, Lepori N, et al. Risk of Adverse Pregnancy Outcomes in Women with CKD. J Am Soc Nephrol 2015; 26: 2011-22

[119] Magee LA, von Dadelszen P, Singer J, Lee T, Rey E, Ross S, et al. The

CHIPS Randomized Controlled Trial (Control of Hypertension in Pregnancy Study): Is Severe Hypertension Just an Elevated Blood Pressure? Hypertension 2016; 68: 1153-9

[120] Hofmeyr GJ, Lawrie TA, Atallah AN, Duley L, Torloni MR. Calcium supplementation during pregnancy for preventing hypertensive disorders and related problems. Cochrane Database Syst Rev 2014; 6: CD001059

[121] Rolnik DL, Wright D, Poon LC, O'Gorman N, Syngelaki A, de Paco Matallana C, et al. Aspirin versus Placebo in Pregnancies at High Risk for Preterm Preeclampsia. N Engl J Med 2017; 377: 613-22

[122] Ojeda-Uribe M, Afif N, Dahan E, Sparsa L, Haby C, Sibilia J, et al. Exposure to abatacept or rituximab in the first trimester of pregnancy in three women with autoimmune diseases. Clin Rheumatol 2013; 32: 695-700

[123] Carmichael SL, Shaw GM, Ma C, Werler MM, Rasmussen SA, Lammer EJ, et al. Maternal corticosteroid use and orofacial clefts. Am J Obstet Gynecol 2007; 197: 585 e1-7; discussion 683-4, e1-7

[124] Skuladottir H, Wilcox AJ, Ma C, Lammer EJ, Rasmussen SA, Werler MM, et al. Corticosteroid use and risk of orofacial clefts. Birth Defects Res A Clin Mol Teratol 2014; 100: 499-506

[125] Lightstone L, Hladunewich MA. Lupus Nephritis and Pregnancy: Concerns and Management. Semin Nephrol 2017; 37: 347-53

[126] Rolfo A, Attini R, Nuzzo AM, Piazzese A, Parisi S, Ferraresi M, et al. Chronic kidney disease may be differentially diagnosed from preeclampsia by serum biomarkers. Kidney Int 2013; 83: 177-81

[127] de Jesús GR, Lacerda MI, Rodrigues BC, Dos Santos FC, do Nascimento AP, Porto LC, et al. VEGF, PlGF and sFlt-1 serum levels allow differentiation between active lupus nephritis during pregnancy and preeclampsia. Arthritis Care Res 2020;

[128] Piccoli GB, Daidola G, Attini R, Parisi S, Fassio F, Naretto C, et al. Kidney biopsy in pregnancy: evidence for counseling? A systematic narrative review. BJOG 2013; 120: 412-27

[129] Wiles K, Chappell L, Clark K, Elman L, Hall M, Lightstone L, et al. Clinical practice guideline on pregnancy and renal disease. BMC Nephrol 2019; 20: 401

[130] Haseler E, Melhem N, Sinha MD. Renal disease in pregnancy: Fetal, neonatal and long-term outcomes. Best Pract Res Clin Obstet Gynaecol 2019; 57: 60-76

[131] Redman CW. Hypertension in pregnancy: the NICE guidelines. Heart 2011; 97: 1967-9

[132] Lamont MC, McDermott C, Thomson AJ, Greer IA. United Kingdom recommendations for obstetric venous thromboembolism prophylaxis: Evidence and rationale. Semin Perinatol 2019; 43: 222-8

[133] Pillay C, Clark K. Postpartum care of women with renal disease. Best Pract Res Clin Obstet Gynaecol 2019; 57: 89-105

[134] Morales E, Galindo M, Trujillo H, Praga M. Update on Lupus Nephritis: Looking for a New Vision. Nephron. 2020:1-13.

[135] Naveed A, Nilubol C, Melancon JK, Girlanda R, Johnson L, Javaid B. Preemptive kidney transplantation in systemic lupus erythematosus. Transplant Proc 2011; 43: 3713-4

[136] Chadban SJ, Ahn C, Axelrod DA, Foster BJ, Kasiske BL, Kher V, et al. KDIGO Clinical Practice Guideline on the Evaluation and Management of Candidates for Kidney Transplantation. Transplantation 2020; 104 (4S1 Suppl 1): S11-S103

[137] Plantinga LC, Patzer RE, Drenkard C, Kramer MR, Klein M, Lim SS, et al. Association of time to kidney transplantation with graft failure among U.S. patients with end-stage renal disease due to lupus nephritis. Arthritis Care Res 2015; 67: 571-81

[138] Wong T, Goral *S. lupus* Nephritis and Kidney Transplantation: Where Are We Today? Adv Chronic Kidney Dis 2019; 26: 313-22

[139] Lionaki S, Skalioti C, Boletis JN. Kidney transplantation in patients with systemic lupus erythematosus. World J Transplant 2014; 4: 176-82

[140] Jorgenson MR, Descourouez JL, Singh T, Astor BC, Panzer SE. Malignancy in Renal Transplant Recipients Exposed to Cyclophosphamide Prior to Transplantation for the Treatment of Native Glomerular Disease. Pharmacotherapy 2018; 38: 51-7

[141] Hibberd AD, Trevillian PR, Wlodarczyk JH, Kemp DG, Stein AM, Gillies AH, et al. Effect of immunosuppression for primary renal disease on the risk of cancer in subsequent renal transplantation: a population-based retrospective cohort study. Transplantation 2013; 95: 122-7

[142] Song L, Wang Y, Zhang J, Song N, Xu X, Lu Y. The risks of cancer development in systemic lupus erythematosus (SLE) patients: a systematic review and meta-analysis. Arthritis Res Ther 2018; 20: 270

[143] Ketteler M, Block GA, Evenepoel P, Fukagawa M, Herzog CA, McCann L, et al. Executive summary of the 2017 KDIGO Chronic Kidney Disease-Mineral and Bone Disorder (CKD-MBD) Guideline Update: what's changed and why it matters. Kidney Int 2017; 92: 26-36

Section 3

Lupus and the Endocrinal System

Chapter 4

Endocrine Manifestations of Systemic Lupus Erythematosus

Ifigenia Kostoglou-Athanassiou, Lambros Athanassiou and Panagiotis Athanassiou

Abstract

Systemic lupus erythematosus (SLE) is a systemic autoimmune disease affecting all organ systems. It affects primarily female patients in the reproductive age. The disease has a variable course from very mild to severe and may be fatal. It is characterized by exacerbations of disease activity called flares. Estrogens seem to be involved in SLE pathogenesis as they have multiple immunomodulating properties. In SLE the autoimmune process affects the neuroendocrine axis. Stress modulates disease expression in lupus patients. The disease affects the endocrine system. Hypothyroidism occurs in SLE patients in a higher rate than that of the general population. Hyperthyroidism is also observed in SLE, however, in the rate expected for the general population. Hashimoto's thyroiditis is observed in SLE in a higher rate than that of the general population. Hyperparathyroidism is also observed in SLE, primary and secondary in the context of renal insufficiency due to lupus nephritis. Addison's disease is rare in SLE. Cushing's disease due to an adrenal adenoma has been observed, but it is rare. Ovarian function may be compromised in SLE, due to autoimmune oophoritis or drug toxicity. The recognition of endocrine disease in SLE is important as it may guide proper management and symptom amelioration.

Keywords: systemic lupus erythematosus, estrogens, neuroendocrine axis, stress, hypothyroidism, hyperthyroidism, Hashimoto's thyroiditis, hyperparathyroidism, ovarian function

1. Introduction

Systemic lupus erythematosus (SLE) is a systemic autoimmune disease affecting all organ systems [1]. It affects mainly joints, skin, blood vessels, heart, lung, kidneys, liver and the nervous system [2]. It is the prototype of systemic autoimmune diseases. In patients with SLE the immune system attacks tissues and cells leading to inflammation and damage [3]. The course of SLE is variable, and maybe either mild or severe leading sometimes to fatal damage and death [4]. The disease is characterized by periods of exacerbation, which are called flares and periods of remission [5]. SLE occurs nine times more often in the female gender mainly in the reproductive age, and it is more frequent in people of non-European descent [6]. Different types of autoantibodies are present in SLE patients [7]. The B lymphocyte is believed to play a major pathogenic role in the disease and many different autoantibodies are detected, therefore the disease is classified as a "B-cell disease" [8, 9]. However, T lymphocytes also play a role in the immunopathogenesis of SLE [10]. Because of the presence of

IntechOpen

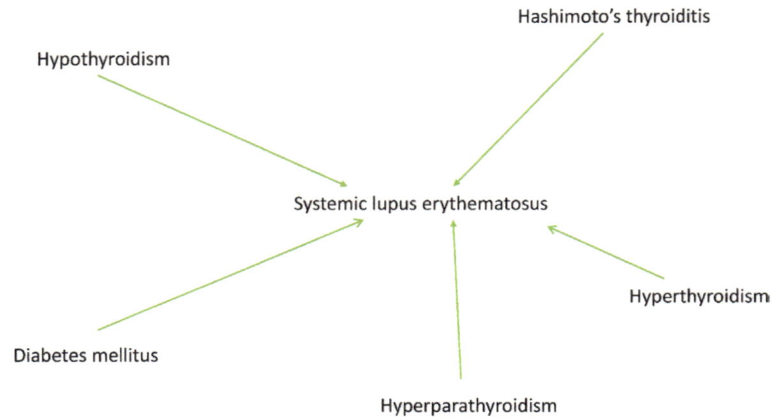

Figure 1.
Common endocrine disorders in systemic lupus erythematosus.

many different autoantibodies, SLE is classified as a "B-cell disease." Patients with SLE present with symptoms and inflammatory involvement that can affect virtually every organ [11]. The main features of SLE include the production of antinuclear antibodies and the deposition of immune complexes in basement membranes throughout the body where they induce an inflammatory response [12, 13]. Genetic, epigenetic, and environmental factors contribute to the development of this autoimmune process. Endocrine manifestations as expected also occur in patients with systemic lupus erythematosus [14] (**Figure 1**). Hypothyroidism has been observed in a higher rate than that expected in the general population. Hyperthyroidism has also been observed. Autoimmune Hashimoto's thyroiditis has been observed in a higher rate than that expected in the general population. Graves' disease has been observed in patients with SLE. Hyperparathyroidism has been observed in patients with SLE, mainly in the context of lupus nephritis. Hypoparathyroidism has also been observed. Autoimmune oophoritis leading to ovarian failure has been observed in patients with SLE. Despite the multisystem nature of the disease, it appears that it respects the adrenals, so that Addison's disease is extremely rare in SLE.

2. The neuroendocrine axis in systemic lupus erythematosus

SLE is a systemic autoimmune disease characterized by a loss of self-tolerance [15]. The immune system is activated in the disease and pro-inflammatory cytokines are secreted [16]. The immune system and the neuroendocrine system are interconnected [17]. The two systems interact in a bidirectional manner (**Figure 2**). During the autoimmune inflammatory response cytokines released from immune cells affect the neuroendocrine axis [18, 19]. In turn the neuroendocrine system secretes hormones which modulate the immune response [20].

The main target of activation by cytokines is the hypothalamic–pituitary–adrenal (HPA) axis. Interleukin (IL) -1a and -1b, IL-6 and tumor necrosis factor (TNF)-a, which are released sequentially from macrophages upon activation, are powerful activators of the HPA axis. In vitro studies in isolated hypothalamic tissue have shown the ability of IL-1a, IL-1b, IL-6, IL-8 and TNF-a to initiate the release of corticotropin-releasing hormone (CRH) [21, 22]. In humans, a blunted HPA axis response to stimulation with hypoglycemia or CRH was shown in several autoimmune diseases, including rheumatoid arthritis, Sjogren's syndrome, fibromyalgia and SLE [23]. However, the relationship between HPA axis reactivity

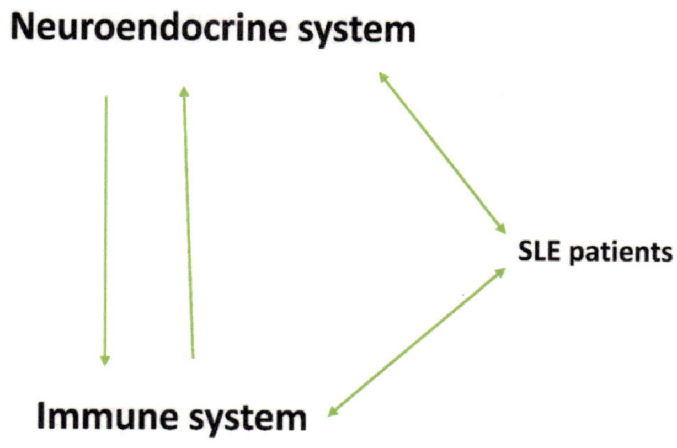

Figure 2.
The interaction between the neuroendocrine and immune systems in systemic lupus erythematosus.

and inflammatory disease was challenged by experiments which showed that in high-stress situations, rats who had a robust corticosterone-response to stress developed more severe inflammation than rats who had a less profound corticosterone response [24]. Differences in the HPA axis response to stress may discriminate patients who seem to have the same disease, but may have different responses to treatment [25]. The HPA axis in important in regulating disease severity in SLE. However, the development of the disease may alter the HPA axis response.

Prolactin (PRL) is a peptide hormone produced by the anterior pituitary. PRL can be produced by lymphocytes, which in turn express PRL receptors [26, 27]. Thus, PRL may have immunomodulatory functions [27–29]. Increased PRL levels have been observed in male and female patients with lupus [30, 31]. Furthermore, suppression of PRL secretion with bromocriptine provides beneficial effects in murine lupus and possibly in lupus patients [32]. Treatment with PRL breaks tolerance and induces a lupus like illness in autoimmune mice. PRL is in effect also a cytokine [29]. PRL receptors are distributed in the immune system [33]. Mild and moderate hyperprolactinemia has been demonstrated in 20–30% of SLE patients and was associated with active disease. Hyperprolactinemia may have a role in lupus nephritis and CNS involvement of patients who have SLE [34]. Elevated PRL levels were associated with increased disease activity in SLE and prolactin may have a pathogenic role in SLE [35]. Thus, PRL, a peptide hormone derived from the anterior pituitary gland and lymphocytes participates in the regulation of the immune response, stimulates immune cells and belongs to a network of immune endocrine interaction. Hyperprolactinemia has been found in SLE and PRL may participate in SLE activation during pregnancy [35]. High levels of prolactin may lead to the development or the exacerbation of an autoimmune disease such as SLE [36]. Prolactin is a bioactive hormone acting both as a hormone as well as a cytokine and it may act as an immunomodulator affecting the negative selection of autoreactive B lymphocytes [29].

2.1 Stress and systemic lupus erythematosus

The adrenergic nervous system runs from the CNS to lymphoid organs, namely the thymus, spleen and lymph nodes. Its effects are mediated by noradrenaline which acts through the relevant receptors [37]. Noradrenaline receptors are expressed by immune cells, namely T and B lymphocytes and macrophages [38]. Noradrenaline and adrenaline stimulate IL-10 and transforming growth factor-b production, thus enhancing Th2 immunity [39, 40]. In SLE, a disease driven by excess IL-10, disease activity may increase during states of high catecholamine release, such as acute stress. In a prospective study of patients with SLE, disease flares were associated with emotional stress or with the number or severity of daily stressors [41, 42]. Additionally, the effect of acute psychological stress induced differential immune response in SLE patients as compared to controls [43].

The hypothalamic–pituitary–adrenal axis responds to inflammatory cytokines [44]. It has been demonstrated that inflammatory cytokines, such as IL-1a and IL-1b, IL-6 and TNF-a are powerful activators of the hypothalamic–pituitary–adrenal axis [45, 46]. In SLE patients with central nervous system involvement elevated levels of inflammatory cytokines were observed in the cerebrospinal fluid [47] suggesting an involvement of these inflammatory cytokines in disease pathogenesis.

2.2 Estrogens in the pathogenesis of systemic lupus erythematosus

SLE is a disease affecting primarily female patients in the reproductive age [48]. Evidence exists implicating estrogens in the pathogenesis of SLE [49]. An extensive cross-talk takes place between estrogen and the immune system. Estrogens are a major modulating factor of the immune response [50] (**Figure 3**). Epidemiological evidence implicates estrogens in the pathogenesis of SLE, as during childhood where estrogen secretion is minimal the female: male ratio is 3:1 as opposed to 9:1 in the reproductive age. In the postmenopausal period the ratio is 8:1 [51]. Evidence has shown that women with early menarche, or treated with oral contraceptives or hormone replacement therapy have an increased risk for SLE [52, 53]. The presence of the X chromosome appears also to be important for the pathogenesis of SLE. There appears to be a gene dose effect, as the prevalence of SLE in Klinefelter's syndrome (XXY) is 14-fold that in the general male population, whereas it is decreased in female patients with Turner's syndrome (XO) [54]. Pregnancy, in which the concentration of estrogens is extremely increased can cause a disease flare or even trigger the development of lupus [55, 56]. The puerperium is characterized by an increased risk for disease relapse [57]. Hormonal factors used for ovulation induction and in vitro fertilization may cause disease flare in SLE [52].

The main pathophysiologic processes of SLE are the loss of self-tolerance and the production of autoantibodies with consequent inflammatory response and organ injury [15]. Estrogens are capable of inducing these alterations in the immune system. Treg cells, immunosuppressive regulatory T cells, play an important role in the maintenance of self-tolerance and the prevention of autoimmunity. SLE

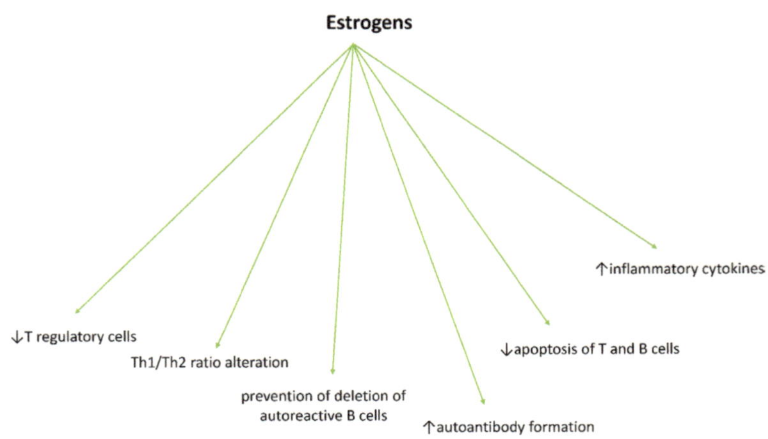

Figure 3.
The effect of estrogens on the immune system.

patients have decreased numbers of Treg cells. Estradiol diminishes Treg cells [52, 58, 59]. In SLE, there is a switch from a type 1 (Th1) to a type 2 (Th2) T cell response where serum levels of Th2 cytokines, such as interleukin 4 (IL-4), IL-6, and IL-10, are elevated and there is decreased production of Th1 cytokines, such as IL-2 and interferon γ [60–62]. Estrogens alter Th1/Th2 ratio thus altering the balance between cellular and humoral immunity. Estrogens induce the development of Th2 lymphocytes and B cell hyperactivity leading to enhanced antibody production [63]. Estrogens promote the life span of lymphocytes by decreasing apoptosis of T and B cells [64]. Thus, estrogens seem to play a key role in the development of autoimmunity. They suppress self-tolerance reducing Treg cells [65]. They alter the Th1/Th2 ratio, favoring the predominance of humoral immunity. They prevent the deletion of autoreactive B cells [66]. They induce the generation of autoantibodies and they stimulate the production of inflammatory cytokines [67].

3. Endocrine disorders in systemic lupus erythematosus

3.1 Thyroid disease in SLE

Autoimmune thyroid disease has been observed in patients with systemic lupus erythematosus, such as autoimmune Hashimoto's thyroiditis, hypothyroidism and Graves' disease.

3.1.1 Hypothyroidism

Hypothyroidism is observed in patients with SLE in a higher rate than in the normal population. In particular, Munoz and Isenberg [14] reported a rate of 5.22% hypothyroidism, i.e. 37 patients, in their cohort of 708 patients with SLE in University College of London Hospital, as compared to 1–2% in the general UK population. In this cohort the onset of hypothyroidism occurred after the onset of SLE oftener. Other reports confirmed a higher than in the general population rate of hypothyroidism in SLE. In particular, Ong and Choy [68] in a Malaysian population of SLE patients observed a prevalence of hypothyroidism of 3.7%. Antonelli et al. [69] reported a prevalence of hypothyroidism of 4.5%. In an earlier report from the University College of London Hospital SLE cohort Pyne and Isenberg [70] reported a prevalence of hypothyroidism of 5.7%.

3.1.2 Hyperthyroidism

Hyperthyroidism is observed in patients with SLE. In their cohort of 708 patients with SLE Munoz and Isenberg [14] observed a prevalence of hyperthyroidism of 1.41% (10/708 SLE patients), similar to that in the general population [71]. Watad *et al* [72] and Ong *et al* [68] reported a prevalence of hyperthyroidism in SLE patients of 2.59% and 2.6%, respectively. Chan *et al* [73] observed a prevalence of 5.8% of hyperthyroidism in a study of 69 SLE patients. However, only 2.9% had a clinical hyperthyroidism.

3.1.3 Autoimmune Hashimoto's thyroiditis

Autoimmune Hashimoto's thyroiditis is frequently observed in patients with SLE. The prevalence of Hashimoto's thyroiditis in patients with SLE as opposed to control subjects was investigated in a study [74]. The association of Hashinoto's Hashimoto's thyroiditis and anti-thyroid antibodies to the clinical, serological profile and disease activity as well as cumulative organ damage in this group was also investigated. In a group of 301 SLE patients and 141 controls TSH levels, T4 levels, antiTg antibodies and antiTPO antibodies were measured by chemiluminescence and immunometric methods. The serological and clinical profile of the patients was reviewed. SLE disease activity was measured using the SLEDAI index. The prevalence of Hashimoto's thyroiditis was 12.6% in SLE as opposed to 5.6% in controls, the difference being statistically significant. A lower prevalence of malar rash and a higher prevalence of anti-Sm was noted in lupus patients with Hashimoto's thyroiditis. No association was noted between Hashimoto's thyroiditis and disease activity of cumulative organ damage. In conclusion, a two-fold increased risk of Hashimoto's thyroiditis was noted in lupus patients. In a study performed in China 63 cases of lupus patients who also had Hashimoto's thyroiditis were studied [75]. Lupus patients were classified in four groups, those in remission, those with low disease activity, those with moderate and those with high disease activity. Free T3 levels were found to be negatively correlated with disease activity. In an effort to find a way to treat effectively Hashimoto's thyroiditis and SLE a group of scientists [76] injected human amniotic epithelial cells in murine models of Hashimoto's thyroiditis and SLE. They observed that levels of antiTg, antiTPO antibodies and TSH levels decreased as well as evidence of tissue destruction within the thyroid decreased. Additionally, the injection of human amniotic epithelial cells induced the disappearance of antidsDNA antibodies and ANA in mice with SLE and improved immunoglobulin profiles. It downregulated the ratio of Th17/Treg cells in both Hashimoto thyroiditis and SLE mice and upregulated the proportion of B10 cells. Human epithelial amniotic cells suppressed the levels of pro-inflammatory cytokines, IL-17A and IFN-γ and enhanced TGF-β in the murine models of Hashimoto's thyroiditis and SLE, thus suggesting a common pathogenic substrate in both diseases.

3.1.4 Graves' disease

Graves' disease is a systemic autoimmune disease with multiple manifestations, affecting the thyroid, the eyes and the skin [77]. Cases of Graves' disease have been described in patients with SLE [78]. The case of a patient with Graves' disease who later developed SLE has been described in the literature [79].

3.2 Pancreatic dysfunction in SLE pathogenesis and form

3.2.1 Diabetes mellitus 1

Cases of diabetes mellitus 1 have been described in SLE. In a cohort of SLE patients in the UK the prevalence of diabetes mellitus 1 was investigated [80]. The coexistence of diabetes mellitus 1, SLE and celiac disease has been described in a young female patient [81]. It appears that diabetes mellitus 1 is rare among SLE patients. However, the risk of developing renal disease, retinal disease and peripheral neuropathy requires careful follow up of the patients. It is also important for the physician to decide which complication is due to lupus or diabetes as the management is different.

3.2.2 Diabetes mellitus 2

Diabetes mellitus type 2 is reported with increasing frequency nowadays [82]. Hence, diabetes mellitus 2 has been reported in patients with SLE. In their cohort of 485 SLE patients Cortes et al. [80] reported 4 patients with diabetes mellitus 2 and two considered to have steroid induced diabetes mellitus. Thus, it appears that diabetes mellitus 2 is infrequent within lupus patients. This may be due to the fact, that lupus develops in a younger age than diabetes mellitus 2 [14]. The relationship between SLE and gestational diabetes has been studied in a meta-analysis [83]. It was found that SLE does not seem to increase the risk of gestational diabetes. However, steroid use in SLE may increase the risk of gestational diabetes.

3.3 Parathyroid disease in SLE

3.3.1 Hyperparathyroidism

Primary hyperparathyroidism is frequently recognized nowadays due to the routine measurement of serum calcium levels. Primary hyperparathyroidism has been reported in patients with lupus. However, there are just a few case reports in the literature of patients with SLE and primary hyperparathyroidism. Primary hyperparathyroidism due to the presence of a parathyroid adenoma in a 47-year old female patient with SLE has been described [84]. Hypercalcemia resolved in this patient after removal of the adenoma. Primary hyperparathyroidism due to a cystic parathyroid adenoma has also been described in a 62-year old female patient with SLE [85]. In their cohort of 708 lupus patients Munoz and Isenberg [14] also identified 5 (0.70%) patients with hyperparathyroidism, 1 with primary hyperparathyroidism and 4 patients with secondary hyperparathyroidism in the context of chronic renal failure due to lupus nephritis. Hyperparathyroidism presented after lupus in all cases described.

3.4 Adrenal disease in SLE

3.4.1 Addison's disease

Addison's disease has been reported in patients with SLE. However, there are only a few case reports of Addison's disease in patients with SLE. The case of a 29-year old female patient who presented with Addisonian crisis in the presence of SLE and responded therapeutically to corticosteroids, both as far as Addison's and lupus is concerned has been described [86]. In their cohort of lupus patients Munoz and Isenberg [14] did not identify any patient with Addison's disease. It appears that Addison's disease is a rare occurrence in lupus patients.

3.4.2 Cushing's syndrome

The occurrence of Cushing's syndrome due to an adrenal adenoma in patients with SLE is rare. The case of an 18-year old female patient with subclinical Cushing's syndrome who developed lupus has been described [87]. The patient was successfully treated by surgical removal of the adrenal adenoma. A case of a 51-year old woman with SLE who developed Cushing's syndrome and was found to have a left adrenal adenoma has been described [88]. The patient was successfully managed by laparascopic left adrenalectomy.

4. Ovarian function

Reproductive function of young female patients with SLE is commonly perturbed by various pathophysiologic mechanisms [89]. Ovarian reserve is diminished even in the presence of mild lupus suggesting a direct effect of the disease itself on ovarian function [90, 91] (**Figure 4**). It is possible that the underlying process is autoimmune oophoritis [92–94]. The clinical manifestations of these abnormalities are menstrual irregularity, amenorrhea, or premature ovarian failure. Menstrual irregularities are frequently observed in patients with SLE, and many of them are associated with the activity of the disease [95]. SLE itself induces dysfunction in the hypothalamic–pituitary-ovarian axis and elevates serum prolactin [35, 96, 97]. A study compared the levels of anti–müllerian hormone (AMH) as a marker of ovarian reserve between SLE patients and control subjects and found that SLE patients had significantly lower AMH levels than did the control subjects. No correlation was observed between disease activity and AMH levels [91]. Female SLE patients may have subfertility issues due to active disease, the use of immunosuppressive medications and delayed childbearing [98]. These findings show that SLE itself has a negative influence on ovarian reserve and function.

SLE patients presenting with severe manifestations of the disease are treated with the alkylating agent cyclophosphamide [99, 100]. Cyclophosphamide is toxic to the ovaries [101–103]. SLE patients exposed to cyclophosphamide have a much higher risk of developing premature ovarian failure and infertility as compared to those receiving less toxic agents [91, 95, 104]. Cyclophosphamide leads to a decrease in reproductive life span and possibly premature ovarian failure. If the loss of ovarian function develops during or shortly after the completion of therapy, it is termed acute ovarian failure. For those who retain ovarian function after the completion of chemotherapy, a subset will go on to develop premature menopause before the age of 40 [105]. The clinical manifestations of ovarian damage in women at reproductive age vary from temporary irregular menses to amenorrhea, infertility, and premature ovarian failure depending on the magnitude of the damage. The probability of developing permanent ovarian failure depends on the following factors: patient's age and the type, dose, and duration of the treatment. If the patient is older and her ovarian reserve is low, they are less likely to retain or regain menstrual function than younger ones. Studies have documented that cyclophosphamide administration is the most significant risk factor for ovarian failure and that AMH is a sensitive and reliable marker of ovarian reserve and damage after exposure to cyclophosphamide in female patients with SLE [106–108]. In the case of cyclophosphamide administration in lupus patients fertility preservation may be attempted [108]. Currently, embryo or oocyte freezing are the established methods used for fertility preservation in patients receiving gonadotoxic treatment [109–111]. Other

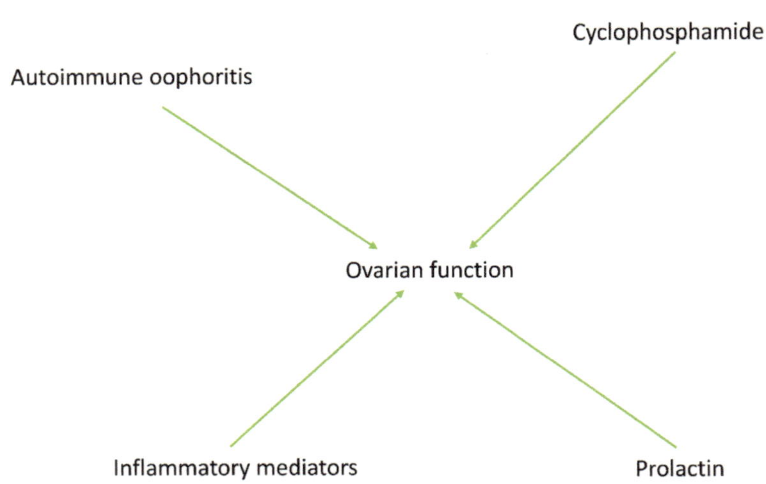

Figure 4.
Factors adversely affecting ovarian function in systemic lupus erythematosus.

options are ovarian tissue freezing and the use of gonadotropin-releasing (GnRH) hormone agonist treatment concurrently with chemotherapy [112, 113].

In conclusion, the reproductive function of female SLE patients can be adversely affected by various mechanisms such as, the chronic inflammatory state, autoimmune ovarian disease in the form of autoimmune oophoritis, lupus flares associated with hyperprolactinemia, which may interfere with ovulation and may modulate immune activity and temporary or even permanent premature ovarian failure as a result of the administration of cytotoxic agents such as cyclophosphamide.

5. Conclusion

SLE is a systemic autoimmune disease which affects all organ systems and occurs frequently in female patients in the reproductive period. Estrogens appear to modulate the immune response, induce loss of self-tolerance, alter the Th1/Th2 balance in favor of the Th2 process, induce the survival of T and B lymphocytes and the production of autoantibodies. Estrogens appear to be involved in the pathogenesis of SLE. In SLE neuroendocrine system function is affected by the autoimmune process, the neuroendocrine system affecting in turn the disease process. Stress appears to affect disease expression in lupus patients. In SLE hypothyroidism occurs oftener than in the general population, hyperthyroidism occurs in the same rate as in the general population and Hashimoto's thyroiditis is present oftener than in a control population. Diabetes mellitus 1 occurs sometimes, diabetes mellitus 2 occurs less frequently than in the general population. Hyperparathyroidism has been observed in lupus patients. Addison's disease is extremely rare in lupus patients. Cushing's disease occurs infrequently in lupus patients. The ovarian function is affected in female SLE patients. Primary ovarian failure may occur due to autoimmune oophoritis. Cyclophosphamide in SLE is used and its use may be accompanied by the development of premature ovarian failure. The recognition of endocrine disease is important in SLE as symptoms may be similar to those of lupus, however management may be different. The recognition and treatment of an endocrine problem in SLE may guide treatment and lead to symptom amelioration and proper patient management.

Author details

Ifigenia Kostoglou-Athanassiou[1]*, Lambros Athanassiou[2] and Panagiotis Athanassiou[3]

1 Department of Endocrinology, Asclepeion Hospital, Voula, Athens, Greece

2 Department of Rheumatology, Asclepeion Hospital, Voula, Athens, Greece

3 Department of Rheumatology, St. Paul's Hospital, Thessaloniki, Greece

*Address all correspondence to: ikostoglouathanassiou@yahoo.gr

References

[1] Aringer M, Costenbader K, Daikh D, et al. 2019 European League Against Rheumatism/American College of Rheumatology classification criteria for systemic lupus erythematosus. Ann Rheum Dis. Sep 2019;78(9):1151-1159. doi:10.1136/annrheumdis-2018-214819

[2] Fava A, Petri M. Systemic lupus erythematosus: Diagnosis and clinical management. *J Autoimmun*. Jan 2019;96:1-13. doi:10.1016/j.jaut.2018.11.001

[3] Durcan L, O'Dwyer T, Petri M. Management strategies and future directions for systemic lupus erythematosus in adults. *Lancet*. Jun 8 2019;393(10188):2332-2343. doi:10.1016/s0140-6736(19)30237-5

[4] Tselios K, Gladman DD, Touma Z, Su J, Anderson N, Urowitz MB. Disease course patterns in systemic lupus erythematosus. *Lupus*. Jan 2019;28(1):114-122. doi:10.1177/0961203318817132

[5] Schäfer VS, Weiß K, Krause A, Schmidt WA. Does erythrocyte sedimentation rate reflect and discriminate flare from infection in systemic lupus erythematosus? Correlation with clinical and laboratory parameters of disease activity. *Clin Rheumatol*. Jul 2018;37(7):1835-1844. doi:10.1007/s10067-018-4093-3

[6] Gergianaki I, Bortoluzzi A, Bertsias G. Update on the epidemiology, risk factors, and disease outcomes of systemic lupus erythematosus. *Best Pract Res Clin Rheumatol*. Apr 2018;32(2):188-205. doi:10.1016/j.berh.2018.09.004

[7] Tipton CM, Hom JR, Fucile CF, Rosenberg AF, Sanz I. Understanding B-cell activation and autoantibody repertoire selection in systemic lupus erythematosus: A B-cell immunomics approach. *Immunol Rev*. Jul 2018;284(1):120-131. doi:10.1111/imr.12660

[8] Yap DYH, Chan TM. B Cell Abnormalities in Systemic Lupus Erythematosus and Lupus Nephritis-Role in Pathogenesis and Effect of Immunosuppressive Treatments. *Int J Mol Sci*. Dec 10 2019;20(24)doi:10.3390/ijms20246231

[9] Ma K, Du W, Wang X, et al. Multiple Functions of B Cells in the Pathogenesis of Systemic Lupus Erythematosus. *Int J Mol Sci*. Nov 29 2019;20(23)doi:10.3390/ijms20236021

[10] Makiyama A, Chiba A, Noto D, et al. Expanded circulating peripheral helper T cells in systemic lupus erythematosus: association with disease activity and B cell differentiation. *Rheumatology (Oxford)*. Oct 1 2019;58(10):1861-1869. doi:10.1093/rheumatology/kez077

[11] Cervera R, Khamashta MA, Font J, et al. Morbidity and mortality in systemic lupus erythematosus during a 10-year period: a comparison of early and late manifestations in a cohort of 1,000 patients. *Medicine (Baltimore)*. Sep 2003;82(5):299-308. doi:10.1097/01.md.0000091181.93122.55

[12] Mistry P, Kaplan MJ. Cell death in the pathogenesis of systemic lupus erythematosus and lupus nephritis. *Clin Immunol*. Dec 2017;185:59-73. doi:10.1016/j.clim.2016.08.010

[13] Morel L. Immunometabolism in systemic lupus erythematosus. *Nat Rev Rheumatol*. May 2017;13(5):280-290. doi:10.1038/nrrheum.2017.43

[14] Muñoz C, Isenberg DA. Review of major endocrine abnormalities in patients with systemic lupus erythematosus. *Clin Exp Rheumatol*. Sep-Oct 2019;37(5):791-796.

[15] Tsokos GC, Lo MS, Costa Reis P, Sullivan KE. New insights into the immunopathogenesis of systemic lupus erythematosus. *Nat Rev Rheumatol*. Nov 22 2016;12(12):716-730. doi:10.1038/nrrheum.2016.186

[16] Kalsi JK, Grossman J, Kim J, et al. Peptides from antibodies to DNA elicit cytokine release from peripheral blood mononuclear cells of patients with systemic lupus erythematosus: relation of cytokine pattern to disease duration. *Lupus*. 2004;13(7):490-500. doi:10.1191/0961203303lu1060oa

[17] Ashley NT, Demas GE. Neuroendocrine-immune circuits, phenotypes, and interactions. *Horm Behav*. Jan 2017;87:25-34. doi:10.1016/j.yhbeh.2016.10.004

[18] Kim YK, Na KS, Myint AM, Leonard BE. The role of pro-inflammatory cytokines in neuroinflammation, neurogenesis and the neuroendocrine system in major depression. *Prog Neuropsychopharmacol Biol Psychiatry*. Jan 4 2016;64:277-84. doi:10.1016/j.pnpbp.2015.06.008

[19] Tsagarakis S, Gillies G, Rees LH, Besser M, Grossman A. Interleukin-1 directly stimulates the release of corticotrophin releasing factor from rat hypothalamus. *Neuroendocrinology*. Jan 1989;49(1):98-101. doi:10.1159/000125096

[20] Bellavance MA, Rivest S. The neuroendocrine control of the innate immune system in health and brain diseases. *Immunol Rev*. Jul 2012;248(1):36-55. doi:10.1111/j.1600-065X.2012.01129.x

[21] Turnbull AV, Rivier C. Regulation of the HPA axis by cytokines. *Brain Behav Immun*. Dec 1995;9(4):253-75. doi:10.1006/brbi.1995.1026

[22] Turnbull AV, Rivier CL. Regulation of the hypothalamic-pituitary-adrenal axis by cytokines: actions and mechanisms of action. *Physiol Rev*. Jan 1999;79(1):1-71. doi:10.1152/physrev.1999.79.1.1

[23] Silverman MN, Sternberg EM. Glucocorticoid regulation of inflammation and its functional correlates: from HPA axis to glucocorticoid receptor dysfunction. *Ann N Y Acad Sci*. Jul 2012;1261:55-63. doi:10.1111/j.1749-6632.2012.06633.x

[24] Chover-Gonzalez AJ, Jessop DS, Tejedor-Real P, Gibert-Rahola J, Harbuz MS. Onset and severity of inflammation in rats exposed to the learned helplessness paradigm. *Rheumatology (Oxford)*. Jul 2000;39(7):764-71. doi:10.1093/rheumatology/39.7.764

[25] Harbuz MS, Chover-Gonzalez AJ, Jessop DS. Hypothalamo-pituitary-adrenal axis and chronic immune activation. *Ann N Y Acad Sci*. May 2003;992:99-106. doi:10.1111/j.1749-6632.2003.tb03141.x

[26] Recalde G, Moreno-Sosa T, Yúdica F, et al. Contribution of sex steroids and prolactin to the modulation of T and B cells during autoimmunity. *Autoimmun Rev*. May 2018;17(5):504-512. doi:10.1016/j.autrev.2018.03.006

[27] Saha S, Tieng A, Pepeljugoski KP, Zandamn-Goddard G, Peeva E. Prolactin, systemic lupus erythe matosus, and autoreactive B cells: lessons learnt from murine models. *Clin Rev Allergy Immunol*. Feb 2011;40(1):8-15. doi:10.1007/s12016-009-8182-6

[28] Borba VV, Zandman-Goddard G, Shoenfeld Y. Prolactin and Autoimmunity. *Front Immunol*. 2018;9:73. doi:10.3389/fimmu.2018.00073

[29] Borba VV, Zandman-Goddard G, Shoenfeld Y. Prolactin and autoimmunity: The hormone as an

inflammatory cytokine. *Best Pract Res Clin Endocrinol Metab*. Dec 2019;33(6):101324. doi:10.1016/j.beem.2019.101324

[30] Jacobi AM, Rohde W, Ventz M, Riemekasten G, Burmester GR, Hiepe F. Enhanced serum prolactin (PRL) in patients with systemic lupus erythematosus: PRL levels are related to the disease activity. *Lupus*. 2001;10(8):554-61. doi:10.1191/096120301701549688

[31] Jacobi AM, Rohde W, Volk HD, Dörner T, Burmester GR, Hiepe F. Prolactin enhances the in vitro production of IgG in peripheral blood mononuclear cells from patients with systemic lupus erythematosus but not from healthy controls. *Ann Rheum Dis*. Mar 2001;60(3):242-7. doi:10.1136/ard.60.3.242

[32] Walker SE. Treatment of systemic lupus erythematosus with bromo criptine. *Lupus*. 2001;10(3):197-202. doi:10.1191/096120301666625458

[33] Leite De Moraes MC, Touraine P, Gagnerault MC, Savino W, Kelly PA, Dardenne M. Prolactin receptors and the immune system. *Ann Endocrinol (Paris)*. 1995;56(6):567-70.

[34] Vera-Lastra O, Jara LJ, Espinoza LR. Prolactin and autoimmunity. *Autoimmun Rev*. Dec 2002;1(6):360-4. doi:10.1016/s1568-9972(02)00081-2

[35] Jara LJ, Medina G, Saavedra MA, et al. Prolactin has a pathogenic role in systemic lupus erythematosus. *Immunol Res*. Apr 2017;65(2):512-523. doi:10.1007/s12026-016-8891-x

[36] Vieira Borba V, Sharif K, Shoenfeld Y. Breastfeeding and autoimmunity: Programing health from the beginning. *Am J Reprod Immunol*. Jan 2018;79(1)doi:10.1111/aji.12778

[37] Elenkov IJ, Wilder RL, Chrousos GP, Vizi ES. The sympathetic nerve--an integrative interface between two supersystems: the brain and the immune system. *Pharmacol Rev*. Dec 2000;52(4):595-638.

[38] Sharma D, Farrar JD. Adrenergic regulation of immune cell function and inflammation. *Semin Immunopathol*. Dec 2020;42(6):709-717. doi:10.1007/s00281-020-00829-6

[39] Elenkov IJ, Papanicolaou DA, Wilder RL, Chrousos GP. Modulatory effects of glucocorticoids and catecholamines on human interleukin-12 and interleukin-10 production: clinical implications. *Proc Assoc Am Physicians*. Sep 1996;108(5):374-81.

[40] Elenkov IJ, Chrousos GP, Wilder RL. Neuroendocrine regulation of IL-12 and TNF-alpha/IL-10 balance. Clinical implications. *Ann N Y Acad Sci*. 2000;917:94-105. doi:10.1111/j.1749-6632.2000.tb05374.x

[41] Da Costa D, Dobkin PL, Pinard L, et al. The role of stress in functional disability among women with systemic lupus erythematosus: a prospective study. *Arthritis Care Res*. Apr 1999;12(2):112-9. doi:10.1002/1529-0131(199904)12:2<112::aid-art6>3.0.co;2-2

[42] Pawlak CR, Witte T, Heiken H, et al. Flares in patients with systemic lupus erythematosus are associated with daily psychological stress. *Psychother Psychosom*. May-Jun 2003;72(3):159-65. doi:10.1159/000069735

[43] Pawlak CR, Jacobs R, Mikeska E, et al. Patients with systemic lupus erythematosus differ from healthy controls in their immunological response to acute psychological stress. *Brain Behav Immun*. Dec 1999;13(4):287-302. doi:10.1006/brbi.1999.0553

[44] Szyper-Kravitz M, Zandman-Goddard G, Lahita RG, Shoenfeld Y. The neuroendocrine-immune interactions in systemic lupus erythematosus: a basis for understanding disease pathogenesis and complexity. *Rheum Dis Clin North Am*. Feb 2005;31(1):161-75, x. doi:10.1016/j.rdc.2004.10.004

[45] Yasin SA, Costa A, Forsling ML, Grossman A. Interleukin-1 beta and interleukin-6 stimulate neurohypo physial hormone release in vitro. *J Neuroendocrinol*. Apr 1994;6(2):179-84. doi:10.1111/j.1365-2826.1994.tb00570.x

[46] Kostoglou-Athanassiou I, Costa A, Navarra P, Nappi G, Forsling ML, Grossman AB. Endotoxin stimulates an endogenous pathway regulating corticotropin-releasing hormone and vasopressin release involving the generation of nitric oxide and carbon monoxide. Article. *Journal of Neuroimmunology*. Jun 1998;86(1):104-109. doi:10.1016/s0165-5728(98)00028-9

[47] Baraczka K, Nékám K, Pozsonyi T, Szüts I, Ormos G. Investigation of cytokine (tumor necrosis factor-alpha, interleukin-6, interleukin-10) concentrations in the cerebrospinal fluid of female patients with multiple sclerosis and systemic lupus erythematosus. *Eur J Neurol*. Jan 2004;11(1):37-42. doi:10.1046/j.1351-5101.2003.00706.x

[48] Margery-Muir AA, Bundell C, Nelson D, Groth DM, Wetherall JD. Gender balance in patients with systemic lupus erythematosus. *Autoimmun Rev*. Mar 2017;16(3):258-268. doi:10.1016/j.autrev.2017.01.007

[49] Lahita RG. The importance of estrogens in systemic lupus erythematosus. *Clin Immunol Immunopathol*. Apr 1992;63(1):17-8. doi:10.1016/0090-1229(92)90086-4

[50] Cutolo M, Capellino S, Sulli A, et al. Estrogens and autoimmune diseases. *Ann N Y Acad Sci*. Nov 2006;1089:538-47. doi:10.1196/annals.1386.043

[51] Lahita RG. The role of sex hormones in systemic lupus erythematosus. *Curr Opin Rheumatol*. Sep 1999;11(5):352-6. doi:10.1097/00002281-199909000-00005

[52] Costenbader KH, Feskanich D, Stampfer MJ, Karlson EW. Reproductive and menopausal factors and risk of systemic lupus erythematosus in women. *Arthritis Rheum*. Apr 2007;56(4):1251-62. doi:10.1002/art.22510

[53] Buyon JP, Petri MA, Kim MY, et al. The effect of combined estrogen and progesterone hormone replacement therapy on disease activity in systemic lupus erythematosus: a randomized trial. *Ann Intern Med*. Jun 21 2005;142(12 Pt 1):953-62. doi:10.7326/0003-4819-142-12_part_1-200506210-00004

[54] Scofield RH, Bruner GR, Namjou B, et al. Klinefelter's syndrome (47,XXY) in male systemic lupus erythematosus patients: support for the notion of a gene-dose effect from the X chromosome. *Arthritis Rheum*. Aug 2008;58(8):2511-7. doi:10.1002/art.23701

[55] Lateef A, Petri M. Systemic Lupus Erythematosus and Pregnancy. *Rheum Dis Clin North Am*. May 2017;43(2):215-226. doi:10.1016/j.rdc.2016.12.009

[56] Eudy AM, Siega-Riz AM, Engel SM, et al. Effect of pregnancy on disease flares in patients with systemic lupus erythematosus. *Ann Rheum Dis*. Jun 2018;77(6):855-860. doi:10.1136/annrheumdis-2017-212535

[57] Stojan G, Baer AN. Flares of systemic lupus erythematosus during pregnancy and the puerperium:

prevention, diagnosis and management. *Expert Rev Clin Immunol*. Jul 2012;8(5):439-53. doi:10.1586/eci.12.36

[58] Lourenço EV, La Cava A. Cytokines in systemic lupus erythematosus. *Curr Mol Med*. Apr 2009;9(3):242-54. doi:10.2174/156652409787847263

[59] Luo CY, Wang L, Sun C, Li DJ. Estrogen enhances the functions of CD4(+)CD25(+)Foxp3(+) regulatory T cells that suppress osteoclast differentiation and bone resorption in vitro. *Cell Mol Immunol*. Jan 2011;8(1):50-8. doi:10.1038/cmi.2010.54

[60] Liblau RS, Singer SM, McDevitt HO. Th1 and Th2 CD4+ T cells in the pathogenesis of organ-specific autoimmune diseases. *Immunol Today*. Jan 1995;16(1):34-8. doi:10.1016/0167-5699(95)80068-9

[61] Constant SL, Bottomly K. Induction of Th1 and Th2 CD4+ T cell responses: the alternative approaches. *Annu Rev Immunol*. 1997;15:297-322. doi:10.1146/annurev.immunol.15.1.297

[62] Street NE, Mosmann TR. Functional diversity of T lymphocytes due to secretion of different cytokine patterns. *Faseb j*. Feb 1991;5(2):171-7. doi:10.1096/fasebj.5.2.1825981

[63] Kanda N, Tsuchida T, Tamaki K. Estrogen enhancement of anti-double-stranded DNA antibody and immunoglobulin G production in peripheral blood mononuclear cells from patients with systemic lupus erythematosus. *Arthritis Rheum*. Feb 1999;42(2):328-37. doi:10.1002/1529-0131(199902)42:2<328::aid-anr16>3.0.co;2-#

[64] Kim WU, Min SY, Hwang SH, Yoo SA, Kim KJ, Cho CS. Effect of oestrogen on T cell apoptosis in patients with systemic lupus erythematosus. *Clin Exp Immunol*. Sep 2010;161(3):453-8. doi:10.1111/j.1365-2249.2010.04194.x

[65] Polanczyk MJ, Hopke C, Vandenbark AA, Offner H. Estrogen-mediated immunomodulation involves reduced activation of effector T cells, potentiation of Treg cells, and enhanced expression of the PD-1 costimulatory pathway. *J Neurosci Res*. Aug 1 2006;84(2):370-8. doi:10.1002/jnr.20881

[66] Seto K, Hoang M, Santos T, Bandyopadhyay M, Kindy MS, Dasgupta S. Non-genomic oestrogen receptor signal in B lymphocytes: An approach towards therapeutic interventions for infection, autoimmunity and cancer. *Int J Biochem Cell Biol*. Jul 2016;76:115-8. doi:10.1016/j.biocel.2016.04.018

[67] Liao ZH, Huang T, Xiao JW, et al. Estrogen signaling effects on muscle-specific immune responses through controlling the recruitment and function of macrophages and T cells. *Skelet Muscle*. Jul 29 2019;9(1):20. doi:10.1186/s13395-019-0205-2

[68] Ong SG, Choy CH. Autoimmune thyroid disease in a cohort of Malaysian SLE patients: frequency, clinical and immunological associations. *Lupus*. Jan 2016;25(1):67-74. doi:10.1177/0961203315593164

[69] Antonelli A, Fallahi P, Mosca M, et al. Prevalence of thyroid dysfunctions in systemic lupus erythematosus. *Metabolism*. Jun 2010;59(6):896-900. doi:10.1016/j.metabol.2009.10.010

[70] Pyne D, Isenberg DA. Autoimmune thyroid disease in systemic lupus erythematosus. *Ann Rheum Dis*. Jan 2002;61(1):70-2. doi:10.1136/ard.61.1.70

[71] Vanderpump MP. The epidemiology of thyroid disease. *Br Med Bull*. 2011;99:39-51. doi:10.1093/bmb/ldr030

[72] Watad A, Mahroum N, Whitby A, et al. Hypothyroidism among SLE patients: Case-control study. *Autoimmun*

Rev. May 2016;15(5):484-6. doi:10.1016/j.autrev.2016.01.019

[73] Chan AT, Al-Saffar Z, Bucknall RC. Thyroid disease in systemic lupus erythematosus and rheumatoid arthritis. *Rheumatology (Oxford)*. Mar 2001;40(3):353-4. doi:10.1093/rheumatology/40.3.353

[74] Posselt RT, Coelho VN, Skare TL. Hashimoto thyroiditis, anti-thyroid antibodies and systemic lupus erythematosus. *Int J Rheum Dis*. Jan 2018;21(1):186-193. doi:10.1111/1756-185x.13089

[75] Liu H, Yang LH, Yin G, Xie QB. [Correlation of Thyroid Autoantibodies,System Lupus Erythematosus Immunologic Indicators and Disease Activity in SLE with HT]. *Sichuan Da Xue Xue Bao Yi Xue Ban*. Mar 2018;49(2):179-182.

[76] Tan B, Yuan W, Li J, et al. Therapeutic effect of human amniotic epithelial cells in murine models of Hashimoto's thyroiditis and Systemic lupus erythematosus. *Cytotherapy*. Oct 2018;20(10):1247-1258. doi:10.1016/j.jcyt.2018.04.001

[77] Smith TJ, Hegedüs L. Graves' Disease. *N Engl J Med*. Oct 20 2016;375(16):1552-1565. doi:10.1056/NEJMra1510030

[78] Ferrari SM, Elia G, Virili C, Centanni M, Antonelli A, Fallahi P. Systemic Lupus Erythematosus and Thyroid Autoimmunity. *Front Endocrinol (Lausanne)*. 2017;8:138. doi:10.3389/fendo.2017.00138

[79] Zhanga Y, Xiaoa X, Haoa Q, Lia X, Renb J, Hu Z. The onset of systemic lupus erythematosus and thyroid dysfunction following Graves' disease – A case report and literature review. *Srp Arh Celok Lek*. Nov-Dec 2016;144(11-12):639-44. doi:10.2298/sarh1612639z

[80] Cortes S, Chambers S, Jerónimo A, Isenberg D. Diabetes mellitus complicating systemic lupus erythematosus - analysis of the UCL lupus cohort and review of the literature. *Lupus*. Nov 2008;17(11):977-80. doi:10.1177/0961203308091539

[81] Zeglaoui H, Landolsi H, Mankai A, Ghedira I, Bouajina E. Type 1 diabetes mellitus, celiac disease, systemic lupus erythematosus and systemic scleroderma in a 15-year-old girl. *Rheumatol Int*. Apr 2010;30(6):793-5. doi:10.1007/s00296-009-0988-2

[82] Wu Y, Ding Y, Tanaka Y, Zhang W. Risk factors contributing to type 2 diabetes and recent advances in the treatment and prevention. *Int J Med Sci*. 2014;11(11):1185-200. doi:10.7150/ijms.10001

[83] Dong Y, Dai Z, Wang Z, et al. Risk of gestational diabetes mellitus in systemic lupus erythematosus pregnancy: a systematic review and meta-analysis. *BMC Pregnancy Childbirth*. May 22 2019;19(1):179. doi:10.1186/s12884-019-2329-0

[84] Galrão LD, Lima IV, Santos L, Santiago MB. [Primary hyperpara thyroidism in a patient with systemic lupus erythematosus]. *Arq Bras Endocrinol Metabol*. Aug 2004;48(4):555-8. Hiperparatireoidismo primário em paciente com lúpus eritematoso sistêmico. doi:10.1590/s0004-27302004000400017

[85] Jiang J, Zhang M, He R, Shen M, Liu W. Functional parathyroid cyst in a patient with systemic lupus erythematosus: a case report. *Endocrinol Diabetes Metab Case Rep*. 2015;2015:140100. doi:10.1530/edm-14-0100

[86] Godswill OC, Odigie OO. Primary Adrenal Insufficiency (Addison's Disease) Associated with Systemic Lupus Erythematosus: A Rare

Occurrence. *Int J Prev Med*. 2014:1324-7. vol. 10.

[87] Nakayama Y, Taura D, Shibue K, Kuramoto N, Mimori T, Inagaki N. A case of systemic lupus erythematosus complicated by subclinical Cushing's syndrome: case report. *Mod Rheumatol Case Rep*. Jan 2020;4(1):16-20. doi:10.1080/24725625.2019.1638049

[88] Shimizu M, Kawata M, Okada T, et al. Concomitant Cushing's syndrome due to adrenal adenoma in a patient with systemic lupus erythematosus. *Intern Med*. Nov 2002;41(11):1044-6. doi:10.2169/internalmedicine.41.1044

[89] Oktem O, Guzel Y, Aksoy S, Aydin E, Urman B. Ovarian function and reproductive outcomes of female patients with systemic lupus erythematosus and the strategies to preserve their fertility. *Obstet Gynecol Surv*. Mar 2015;70(3):196-210. doi:10.1097/ogx.0000000000000160

[90] Medeiros PB, Febrônio MV, Bonfá E, Borba EF, Takiuti AD, Silva CA. Menstrual and hormonal alterations in juvenile systemic lupus erythematosus. *Lupus*. Jan 2009;18(1):38-43. doi:10.1177/0961203308094652

[91] Lawrenz B, Henes J, Henes M, et al. Impact of systemic lupus erythematosus on ovarian reserve in premenopausal women: evaluation by using anti-Muellerian hormone. *Lupus*. Oct 2011;20(11):1193-7. doi:10.1177/0961203311409272

[92] LaBarbera AR, Miller MM, Ober C, Rebar RW. Autoimmune etiology in premature ovarian failure. *Am J Reprod Immunol Microbiol*. Mar 1988;16(3):115-22. doi:10.1111/j.1600-0897.1988.tb00180.x

[93] Chang YS, Lai CC, Chen WS, Wang SH, Chou CT, Tsai CY. Protein-losing enteropathy and premature ovarian failure in a young woman with systemic lupus erythematosus. *Lupus*. Oct 2012;21(11):1237-9. doi:10.1177/0961203312449492

[94] Pasoto SG, Viana VS, Mendonca BB, Yoshinari NH, Bonfa E. Anti-corpus luteum antibody: a novel serological marker for ovarian dysfunction in systemic lupus erythematosus? *J Rheumatol*. May 1999;26(5):1087-93.

[95] Shabanova SS, Ananieva LP, Alekberova ZS, Guzov, II. Ovarian function and disease activity in patients with systemic lupus erythematosus. *Clin Exp Rheumatol*. May-Jun 2008;26(3):436-41.

[96] Joob B, Wiwanitkit V. Prolactin and systemic lupus erythematosus. *Immunol Res*. 2017:975. vol. 4.

[97] Song GG, Lee YH. Circulating prolactin level in systemic lupus erythematosus and its correlation with disease activity: a meta-analysis. *Lupus*. Oct 2017;26(12):1260-1268. doi:10.1177/0961203317693094

[98] Nusbaum JS, Mirza I, Shum J, et al. Sex Differences in Systemic Lupus Erythematosus: Epidemiology, Clinical Considerations, and Disease Pathogenesis. *Mayo Clin Proc*. Feb 2020;95(2):384-394. doi:10.1016/j.mayocp.2019.09.012

[99] Petri M. Cyclophosphamide: new approaches for systemic lupus erythematosus. *Lupus*. 2004;13(5):366-71. doi:10.1191/0961203303lu1028oa

[100] Kado R, McCune WJ. Ovarian protection with gonadotropin-releasing hormone agonists during cyclophosphamide therapy in systemic lupus erythematosus. *Best Pract Res Clin Obstet Gynaecol*. Apr 2020;64:97-106. doi:10.1016/j.bpobgyn.2019.10.008

[101] Spears N, Lopes F, Stefansdottir A, et al. Ovarian damage from

chemotherapy and current approaches to its protection. *Hum Reprod Update*. Nov 5 2019;25(6):673-693. doi:10.1093/humupd/dmz027

[102] Luan Y, Edmonds ME, Woodruff TK, Kim SY. Inhibitors of apoptosis protect the ovarian reserve from cyclophosphamide. *J Endocrinol*. Feb 1 2019;240(2):243-256. doi:10.1530/joe-18-0370

[103] Xiong Y, Liu T, Wang S, Chi H, Chen C, Zheng J. Cyclophosphamide promotes the proliferation inhibition of mouse ovarian granulosa cells and premature ovarian failure by activating the lncRNA-Meg3-p53-p66Shc pathway. *Gene*. Jan 5 2017;596:1-8. doi:10.1016/j.gene.2016.10.011

[104] Harward LE, Mitchell K, Pieper C, Copland S, Criscione-Schreiber LG, Clowse ME. The impact of cyclophosphamide on menstruation and pregnancy in women with rheumatologic disease. *Lupus*. Jan 2013;22(1):81-6. doi:10.1177/0961203312468624

[105] Chemaitilly W, Mertens AC, Mitby P, et al. Acute ovarian failure in the childhood cancer survivor study. *J Clin Endocrinol Metab*. May 2006;91(5):1723-8. doi:10.1210/jc.2006-0020

[106] Mok CC, Chan PT, To CH. Anti-müllerian hormone and ovarian reserve in systemic lupus erythematosus. *Arthritis Rheum*. Jan 2013;65(1):206-10. doi:10.1002/art.37719

[107] Appenzeller S, Blatyta PF, Costallat LT. Ovarian failure in SLE patients using pulse cyclophosphamide: comparison of different regimes. *Rheumatol Int*. Apr 2008;28(6):567-71. doi:10.1007/s00296-007-0478-3

[108] Mersereau J, Dooley MA. Gonadal failure with cyclophosphamide therapy for lupus nephritis: advances in fertility preservation. *Rheum Dis Clin North Am*. Feb 2010;36(1):99-108, viii. doi:10.1016/j.rdc.2009.12.010

[109] Rienzi L, Gracia C, Maggiulli R, et al. Oocyte, embryo and blastocyst cryopreservation in ART: systematic review and meta-analysis comparing slow-freezing versus vitrification to produce evidence for the development of global guidance. *Hum Reprod Update*. Mar 1 2017;23(2):139-155. doi:10.1093/humupd/dmw038

[110] Rajabi Z, Aliakbari F, Yazdekhasti H. Female Fertility Preservation, Clinical and Experimental Options. *J Reprod Infertil*. Jul-Sep 2018;19(3):125-132.

[111] Levi-Setti PE, Patrizio P, Scaravelli G. Evolution of human oocyte cryopreservation: slow freezing versus vitrification. *Curr Opin Endocrinol Diabetes Obes*. Dec 2016;23(6):445-450. doi:10.1097/med.0000000000000289

[112] Yding Andersen C, Mamsen LS, Kristensen SG. FERTILITY PRESERVATION: Freezing of ovarian tissue and clinical opportunities. *Reproduction*. Nov 2019;158(5):F27-f34. doi:10.1530/rep-18-0635

[113] Del Mastro L, Lambertini M. Temporary Ovarian Suppression With Gonadotropin-Releasing Hormone Agonist During Chemotherapy for Fertility Preservation: Toward the End of the Debate? *Oncologist*. Nov 2015;20(11):1233-5. doi:10.1634/theoncologist.2015-0373

Section 4

Lupus Pregnancy: An Update on All

Chapter 5

Systemic Lupus Erythematosus Pregnancy

Melissa Fernandes, Vera Bernardino, Anna Taulaigo, Jorge Fernandes, Ana Lladó and Fátima Serrano

Abstract

Systemic Lupus Erythematosus (SLE) is an autoimmune disease of unknown etiology that often affects women during childbearing age. Pregnant women with SLE are considered high-risk patients, with pregnancy outcomes being complicated by high maternal and fetal mortality and morbidity. Obstetric morbidity includes preterm birth, fetal growth restriction (FGR), and neonatal lupus syndromes. Active SLE during conception is a strong predictor of adverse pregnancy outcomes and exacerbations of disease can occur more frequently during gestation. Therefore, management of maternal SLE should include preventive strategies to minimize disease activity and to reduce adverse pregnancy outcomes. Patients with active disease at time of conception have increased risk of flares, like lupus nephritis, imposing a careful differential diagnosis of pre-eclampsia, keeping in mind that physiological changes of pregnancy may mimic a lupus flare. Major complications arise when anti-phospholipid antibodies are present, like recurrent pregnancy loss, stillbirth, FGR, and thrombosis in the mother. A multidisciplinary approach is hence crucial and should be initiated to all women with SLE at childbearing age with an adequate preconception counseling with assessment of risk factors for adverse maternal and fetal outcomes with a tight pregnancy monitoring plan. Although treatment choices are limited during pregnancy, prophylactic anti-aggregation and anticoagulation agents have proven beneficial in reducing thrombotic events and pre-eclampsia related morbidity. Pharmacological therapy should be tailored, allowing better outcomes for both the mother and the baby. Immunosuppressive and immunomodulators, must be effective in controlling disease activity and safe during pregnancy. Hydroxychloroquine is the main therapy for SLE due to its anti-inflammatory and immunomodulatory effects recommended before and during pregnancy and other immunosuppressive drugs (e.g. azathioprine and calcineurin inhibitors) are used to control disease activity in order to improve obstetrical outcomes. Managing a maternal SLE is a challenging task, but an early approach with multidisciplinary team with close monitoring is essential and can improve maternal and fetal outcomes.

Keywords: Systemic Lupus Erythematosus, Pregnancy, Pre-eclampsia, Antiphospholipid Syndrome, Lupus Nephritis, Immunosuppression, Hydroxychloroquine, Neonatal lupus syndrome

IntechOpen

1. Introduction

Systemic lupus erythematosus (SLE) is a chronic multisystem autoimmune disease characterized by production of autoantibodies and polymorphic manifestations of end-organ damage [1, 2]. The disease can manifest itself in many forms and severity, ranging from mild cutaneous and joint involvement, to devastating ocular complications or lethal renal, cardiac and cerebral involvement [3]. SLE is caused by interactions between susceptibility genes and environmental factors, resulting in irreversible loss of immunologic self-tolerance. Its estimated incidence ranges from 0.3 to 23.2 per 100.000 person-years and it mostly affects women, with a female to male ratio as high as 10–15:1 [4, 5]. In women, prevalence varies between 164 to 406/100.000 [6] and most of them are in childbearing age. For these reasons, reproductive health and family planning are issues of utmost importance for physicians managing SLE patients, including internists, rheumatologists, and gynecologists. Even if fertility is not impaired in SLE, pregnancy represents a high-risk period in the disease course, mainly due to serious potential maternal and fetal complications. On the maternal side, risk of flare is increased during pregnancy, and there is risk of pre-eclampsia (PE) and thrombotic complications, especially in women carrying antiphospholipid antibodies (aPL). On the fetal side, fetal growth restriction (FGR) and preterm birth are feared complications, besides the potential harm caused by maternal antibodies, as it is the case of congenital heart block (CHB) and neonatal lupus in women carrying SS-A and SS-B antibodies. Multidisciplinary approach, preconception counseling, pregnancy planning and increased availability of safe drugs in pregnancy and puerperium have contributed to improve both maternal and fetal outcomes.

2. Immunopathogenesis

The immune system is a multidimensional environment with its main role being to protect the host against foreign pathogens and to remove cellular debris without harming the host. The etiology of SLE is multifactorial which leads to a failure to maintain immune tolerance and immune homeostasis manifested by aberrant immune responses against endogenous nuclear and other self-antigens. The pathogenesis of SLE involves various cells and molecules that intervene in apoptosis, innate and adaptive immune responses [7, 8]. This process involves plasma cells migrating to inflamed tissue where they become long-lived plasma cells that make antibodies and contribute to the formation of immune complexes.

2.1 Genetic predisposition and epigenetics contributions

The etiology of SLE still remains unknown, but genetic (e.g. major histocompatibility complex (MHC), interferon regulatory factor 5 (IRF5)) components and environmental factors (e.g. Epstein–Barr Virus (EBV), UV light) play an important role in the pathogenesis of SLE [9].

2.2 Coexistence: the interaction of pregnancy and SLE

The state of pregnancy is a complex and sophisticated one—it requires physiologic adaptions in all maternal systems, including immune and neuroendocrine alterations in the maternal body, in order to adapt and protect the fetus from immunologic attack by the mother [10].

The induction and maintenance of tolerance throughout pregnancy involves many different immunoregulatory cell types, including cells that reside in the decidua, which are recruited to the placenta or proliferate locally in the decidua, as well as cell surface receptors and secreted molecules that orchestrate tolerogenic mechanism [11].

This modulation of the composition and function of the immune-competent cells and immune-modulatory molecules in the maternal system during pregnancy has the ability to enhance and suppress different immune mechanisms to create a balance that protects the fetus, without compromising the mother's defense against infection [10].

In harmony, estrogen cells and regulatory proteins exert their effects on decidual stromal cells and tolerogenic dendritic cells, expand FOXP3+ T regulatory cells (Treg), calibrate the function of the rapidly increasing number of natural killer (NK) cells and downregulate effector T cells. The fetus promotes tolerance to paternal antigens by migration of fetal cells and cell-free fetal DNA to the maternal circulation during normal pregnancy. The fetus is considered a semi-allogeneic graft and to avoid rejection, a tolerogenic state at the feto-maternal interface has to be induced rapidly [12].

In a simple schematic way, the physiologic immune response to pregnancy occurs by: (1) stimulation of B cells which occurs with production of antibodies; (2) T helper (Th) cells participate as co-stimulatory cells, inducing a shift at the Th 1 and Th 2 helper cell level; (3) leading to a predominance of Th 2 cells during pregnancy which also suppresses the response of cytotoxic T cells; (4) the shift towards the Th 2 response leads to suppression of anti-fetal antigen-mediated immune responses; (5) the hormonal system participates in the suppression of cell-mediated immunity, and thus immune tolerance; and (6) a tight cooperation for preventing a response to fetal antigens occurs between the trophoblast and the maternal immune system [13].

2.2.1 T cell responses in normal pregnancy and in lupus pregnancy

In the case of pregnancy associated with SLE, the main immune abnormality involves the function of T regulatory (Treg) cells, as these are limited in number and in their functions [14]. The main purpose of the Treg cells during a normal pregnancy is to ensure immune tolerance to the fetus, and in the case of SLE, the immune system is confronted with a weaken response which cannot ensure the right settings of the product of conception.

Therefore, the problem arises with the number of Treg cells. In a normal pregnancy, the number of Treg cells increases and contrarily decreases in cases of pregnancy loss and pre-eclampsia. On one hand, pregnancy benefits from the contribution of Treg cells, which ensure maternal-fetal tolerance. On the other hand, Treg cells are defective in SLE [15]. It is also possible that this impaired immune tolerance results in complications such as miscarriage, preterm birth or pre-eclampsia. However, in cases of pregnancy associated with inactive SLE, Treg cells might ensure maternal-fetal tolerance because functional Treg cells predominate. This is one of the reasons why women should be in remission prior to pregnancy [13].

The Th 17 cell is a subset of the T helper which is regulated by Treg cells. They possess great plasticity and its function is to produce IL-17 and other interleukins such as IL-21, IL-22, and IL-17F [16]. These cells which mainly produce IL-17A and IL-17F can turn into cells that produce interferon gamma [17]. Th 17 cells have a role in inflammatory processes in autoimmune diseases and abnormal changes in the ratio of Th 17 cells to Treg cells may be related to spontaneous abortion and premature birth [17, 18]. Torricelli et al., found that pregnant women with SLE demonstrated increased levels of IL-17 together with other cytokines, including IL-6, IL-10, and TNF. This may indicate a hyperactive immune system among pregnant women with SLE, and this may be related to the placenta [18].

However, beyond the limited and mal-function of Treg cells, estrogens are also an important part of the immunopathology of SLE, which in pregnancy plays an important part in shaping the immune tolerance.

2.2.2 Estrogens and its role in normal pregnancy versus lupus pregnancy

Estrogens are related to the immune response system and in high concentrations act simultaneously with other reproductive hormones. It is believed to stimulate increased Th2 cytokines during gestation, being a desirable response to normal pregnancy. However, in SLE patient, excessive Th2 responses can lead to increased secretion of IL-17, which may lead to recurrent miscarriages [13, 18]. By promoting Th 2 responses, estrogens in pregnancy tend to worsen Th 2-mediated diseases such as SLE [16, 17]. Torricelli et al., showed high levels of serum IL-17 in pregnant women with SLE [19].

2.2.3 B cell response in normal pregnancy versus in SLE

In SLE, B cells also have an important role in producing antibodies. The B cells participate in maternal immune tolerance to the fetus with secretion of IL-10, which progressively rises during a normal and healthy pregnancy. However, in SLE patients, IL-10 levels are significantly higher at conception and remain elevated throughout pregnancy and postpartum. IL-10 is a pleiotropic cytokine, with both immune stimulatory and immune suppressive functions. Persistent high levels of IL-10 indicate a constitutional overproduction in SLE, resulting in continuous B cell stimulation [12, 13].

3. Pregnancy planning and monitoring in SLE

SLE pregnancies are considered as a high-risk process. The strongest predictor of adverse pregnancy outcomes is an active SLE at time of conception. Patients with active SLE should postpone pregnancy until SLE is under control [20]. In certain cases, pregnancy is contraindicated in patients with severe organ involvement (e.g. severe renal insufficiency or end stage renal disease, congestive heart failure, severe pulmonary fibrosis, and severe pulmonary hypertension) [21]. Women with a past history of thrombotic events have an increased risk for thrombosis during pregnancy and post-partum, and in these cases there should be a switch from warfarin to low molecular weight heparin [22]. Risk stratification should be performed according to the aPL outline, taking into account the type, titer, and persistence of aPL. By doing so, patients can be divided into "high-risk" and "low-risk" profiles and treatment should be given according to each specific case [23]. Women should be started on folic acid preferably 3 months prior to conception; throughout pregnancy, they should be on calcium and vitamin D [24].

Therefore, it is crucial and mandatory the assessment of risk factors for adverse maternal and fetal outcomes in women with SLE who desire to be pregnant – this starts with preconception counseling and implementing appropriate preventive strategies and an individual-tailored monitoring plan before (switch teratogenic medications for non-teratogenic ones, respecting the wash-out of harmful medications, and being in remission for at least 3 to 6 months' prior conception) and during pregnancy [20].

Once pregnancy is confirmed, a monthly routine need to be ensured and should include: doctor appointments and complete blood analyses, including a complete set of autoantibodies, as well as, specific maternal antibodies such as aPL and anti-Ro/SSA. In the case for patients with current or past renal involvement, blood pressure and 24-h urine proteinuria should be monitored regularly [20, 22].

SLE pregnant should be followed after specific protocols for patients at high-risk of developing hypertensive disorders and/or placental insufficiency. Fetal surveillance should be based on biometric and Doppler findings during the third trimester, and particularly distinguish between early and late FGR, helping to better tailor the time of delivery and reduce perinatal morbidity and mortality. Fetal echocardiography is only indicated if there is suspected fetal dysrhythmia or myocarditis, especially in the context of positive maternal anti-Ro/SSA or anti-La/SSB antibodies [20].

4. SLE & other autoimmune diseases

4.1 Presence of antiphospholipid antibodies

The presence of antiphospholipid antibodies (aPL) during pregnancy is associated with significant risk of maternal and fetal adverse events. The prevalence of aPL in SLE is about 12–44% for anticardiolipin (aCL), 15–34% for lupus anticoagulant (LAC) and 10–19% for anti-beta2 glycoprotein I (β2GPI) antibodies [25]. These antibodies are responsible for an autoimmune hypercoagulable state, known as antiphospholipid syndrome (APS). Even though aPL are present in about a half of patients with SLE, only a fraction of these patients develops antiphospholipid syndrome (APS), which manifests as thrombotic and/or obstetric adverse events, mediated by persistent circulating aPL detected by means of three tests: LAC, aCL and β2GPI antibodies, repeated twice with an interval of 12 weeks apart. A different subset of patients, the so-called "aPL carriers", has been described. These are aPL positive individuals without clinical manifestations, that are at high-risk of prematurity, pre-eclampsia, eclampsia, or HELLP (hemolysis, elevated liver enzyme levels, low platelet count) syndrome. The most severe form of APS is catastrophic antiphospholipid syndrome (CAPS) a potentially fatal and rare condition that women may develop during pregnancy. Its diagnosis is challenging and aggressive treatment is crucial in order to save a patient's life [23].

The outcomes of pregnancies in patients with aPL have significantly improved and live birth rates over 80% are achieved nowadays. The management is based on the risk of profile of aPL and/or previous thrombotic and/or obstetric complications.

4.2 Presence of anti-Ro antibodies

Anti-Ro/SSA and/or anti-La/SSB autoantibodies are detected in approximately 40% of patients with SLE. The transplacental passage of maternal IgG antibodies (anti-Ro/SSA and anti-La/SSB) may lead to neonatal lupus in 1–2% of all pregnancies affected by SLE [26].

Congenital Heart Block (CHB) is the most severe manifestation, affecting 2% of pregnancies with positive antibodies (especially anti-Ro/SSA) and without a previous history of complicated pregnancies. This usually manifests between the 18th and 24th weeks of gestation. The risk increases significantly 10 to 15% in patients who have a prior history of another neonate affected with cutaneous lupus and up to 15–20% in those with a prior neonate affected with CHB [27].

5. Pregnancy: physiological changes versus SLE activity

It is crucial to differentiate physiological changes that occur during a normal pregnancy versus pathological conditions, since both situations can have clinical and/or laboratory changes.

In a healthy pregnancy, many clinical manifestations can overlap those of an active SLE – see **Table 1**. Sex hormone levels vary throughout pregnancy, which affect the immune system and can lead to a SLE flare [28]. The hormonal system has receptors for cytokines, immune cells, and lymphatic tissues. In a pregnancy with SLE, the serum levels of gonadotropins and sex steroids differ from the healthy individuals; as there is a decrease of estradiol, cortisol, testosterone, dehydroepiandrosterone and progesterone. Estrogen stimulates, by itself, the maturation of peripheral immune cells, especially Treg cells, that will further promote the immune system tolerance or suppression. In a healthy pregnancy, as explained in point 2.2.1, Treg cells numbers can increase, providing a higher level of fetal tolerance [15, 28]. However, in SLE pregnancy, a reduced number and function of Treg cells has been detected, which can lead to a worse outcome.

It is also known that pregnancy stimulates an increase in blood volume, involving an increase in plasma volume, raising both red-blood cell and white-blood cell volumes [29]. The discrepancy between plasma volume expansion and red-blood cell augmentation will provoke a hemodilution and cause the so-called, "physiological anemia of pregnancy" (normal hemoglobin of >11 g/dL and hematocrit >33% in the 1st and 3rd trimester). This may be caused by an increase in sodium retention, mediated by mineralocorticoid stimulation, that will lead to fluid retention and, subsequently, vasodilatation. During labor, blood volume will increase even further, due to uterine contractions, squeezing blood out of the intervillous space into the main circulation. So, after delivery, retraction of uterus and interruption of placental circulation will raise about 500 mL of blood, acting like an auto-transfusion.

	Pregnancy changes	**SLE activity**
Clinical Features	Facial flush Hyperpigmentation	Photosensitivity Vespertilio
	Palmar erythema Friable mucous membranes	Oral or nasal ulcers
	Arthralgia	Inflammatory arthritis
	Fatigue	Fatigue Lethargy
	Mild peripheral edema	Moderate to severe edema
	Mild resting dyspnea	Pleuritis Pericarditis
Laboratory features	Mild anemia	Immune hemolytic anemia
	Mild thrombocytopenia	Thrombocytopenia Leukopenia Lymphopenia
	Mild ⇧ ESR	⇧ inflammatory marker levels
	Physiologic proteinuria	Proteinuria >300 mg/day
		Active urinary sediment

Abbreviation: ESR - erythrocyte sedimentation rate.

Table 1.
Overlapping features of pregnancy and systemic lupus erythematosus (SLE).

Levels of clotting factors, fibrinogen, platelet production, aggregation and destruction will also be elevated, causing a hypercoagulable state [29]. Endogenous anticoagulants, such as protein S, are also diminished and there is an acquired resistance to activated protein C. Fibrinolysis is also impaired due to placental production of plasminogen activator inhibitor. Overall, these imbalances will also promote a prothrombotic and procoagulant status. This process of enhanced coagulation and increased blood volume guarantees important functions: supplying an increase uterus, a placenta and a growing fetus, and protecting the mother from a massive bleeding during labor [29].

Following delivery, blood volume will then be restored to its normal levels about 8 weeks' post-partum. Moreover, it is known that the increase in blood volume leads to an increase in glomerular filtration, which in turn will stress the renal function [28]. This aggravation will be more pronounced in patients with underlying kidney disease. In a healthy pregnancy, glomerular filtration rate can increase up to 50% and creatinine clearance by 30%. Tubular reabsorption of sodium is then enhanced, but glucose and amino acids may not be absorbed in the same proportion, leading to glycosuria and aminoaciduria in healthy pregnancies [29]. Renal failure before pregnancy, as it may occur un SLE, is related to poor fetal outcome and early delivery [28]. When serum creatinine is higher than 140 mmol/L, there's a 50% chance of miscarriage; this probability raises up to 80% when creatinine is over 400 mmol/L. Nephrotic syndrome will further worsen the prognosis, as it relates to another increased risk of thrombosis.

Cardiac output will increase, reaching a plateau at 28–32 weeks' gestation [29]. Stroke volume will increase ejection fraction and maternal heart rate is also accelerated [30]. However, the distended uterus compresses aortocaval circulation, reducing cardiac filling while in supine position. Filling pressure will not change, due to myocardial remodeling that occurs during pregnancy. Peripheral and systemic vascular resistance is reduced, due to vasodilation. Altogether, these changes will contribute for blood pressure stabilization in a healthy pregnancy. This equilibrium will be imbalanced in nephrotic syndrome and PE situations, as cardiac output and blood pressure are elevated.

The enlarged gravid uterus displaces the heart to the left and upward, so the electrocardiogram may present sinus tachycardia, benign dysrhythmias, depressed ST segments or flattened T waves, left axis deviation and left ventricular hypertrophy [29]. Diaphragm will also be displaced, progressively decreasing functional residual capacity (FRC), expiratory reserve volume and residual volume. Tidal volume and inspiratory reserve volume will increase, so that vital capacity will remain unchanged. Reduction of FRC combined with an increase of oxygen consumption can provoke a rapid development of maternal hypoxemia during apnea.

Heartburn progressively increases, as the uterus displaces and disrupts the lower esophageal sphincter, intensified by progesterone induced relaxation [29]. Although gastric pressure increases, gastric emptying is normal. Obstipation is frequent, due to an increased intestinal transit time. Liver enzymes are normal, but placental production of alkaline phosphatases can increase up to 2–4-fold of its normal range. Gallstone formation can be induced by impaired emptying of gallbladder.

Neuropsychiatric symptoms represent a clinical challenge, as they can result from the pregnancy itself or postpartum period, but also from preeclampsia, eclampsia, or even electrolyte imbalance, infection, renal failure, and drug toxicity [31]. For example, headaches can result from hormonal and postural changes, insomnia, anxiety, preeclampsia, but can also be a symptom of neurolupus [32]. An accurate clinical history and examination is hence always mandatory.

Laboratory tests may reveal different values from the normal range that are considered acceptable in pregnancy, which makes them less reliable. Pregnant women frequently present mild anemia and thrombocytopenia, elevated erythrocyte sedimentation rate, proteinuria (up to 300 mg/day) and increased levels of complement [31]. So, it is essential that a proper evaluation of disease activity is done. Also, complement levels can be falsely increased, so it will not serve as a strong biomarker. On the other hand, anti-DNA antibodies can still be related to disease activity. The scales of pregnancy SLE, as mentioned above, SLEPDAI, LAI-P, and BILAG2004-Pregnancy index, can also be a useful tool, combined with clinical judgment and laboratory parameters.

6. Disease activity assessment during pregnancy

As mentioned above, a strict assessment and control of disease activity before and throughout pregnancy is fundamental. Physiological changes in pregnancy may mimic a lupus flare (e.g. constitutional symptoms, non-inflammatory joint pain, skin rash, alopecia), as well as, laboratory changes (e.g. anemia, thrombocytopenia, proteinuria, increase of ESR and complement levels).

In order to reduce confounding features from physiological pregnancy and SLE exacerbations, three scores were modified in order to adapt to these changes: the SLE-Pregnancy Disease Activity Index (SLEPDAI), the LAI (Lupus Activity Index) in Pregnancy (LAI-P), and the modified SLAM (Systemic Lupus Activity Measure) (m-SLAM). Two other pregnancy-adapted scores have been introduced more recently, the modified-European consensus lupus activity measurement (m-ECLAM) and the British Isles Lupus Assessment Group-2004 for pregnancy (BILAG2004-P).

In all the above-mentioned indices, modifications were made to address influential items: some were eliminated (e.g. ESR, asthenia) and others were adapted to physiological pregnancy changes (e.g. proteinuria levels), emphasizing the need to differentiate those changes from pregnancy comorbidities (e.g. PE/E). The scoring of each index is calculated in the same way as the original version, except for the LAI-P, in which the weighted score given to each item has been modified. Although many attempts have been made to have a reliable tool, the clinical judgment of an experienced physician remains the gold standard in the management of pregnant women with SLE. As recently recommended, these women should be frequently monitored (every 2 to 8 weeks). During each visit, prostaglandin A (PGA) in conjunction with at least one of the activity tools and pregnancy-specific SLE activity indices (such as SLEPDAI, LAI-P, BILAG 2004- P) should be applied [20].

7. Maternal and fetal complications during lupus pregnancy

Maternal and fetal complications are more frequent in lupus pregnancy than in healthy ones. So, even if new treatment strategies have been incorporated in guidelines for managing this complex situation, SLE is still a severe risk factor for pregnancy.

As discussed, SLE pregnancy is related to an increased risk of miscarriage, stillbirth, neonatal death, premature delivery and FGR [33, 34]. Cesarean section due to pregnancy complications is also more prevalent in lupus patients. A large nationwide study revealed that maternal mortality rate in SLE patients reaches 325/100,000 live births, meaning more than 20-fold higher than in non-SLE population [35]. The risk for other maternal complications includes thrombosis, hypertension, infection, thrombocytopenia, and transfusion, being each 3- to 7-fold higher in SLE population. Gestational hypertension, apart from pre-eclampsia, may provoke long-term complications related to cardiovascular and peripheral artery disease [34].

The risk of gestational diabetes is also increased in SLE pregnancy [22, 36]. It is mainly related to glucocorticoid therapy during pregnancy. About 10% of gestational diabetes result from autoimmune activity (GADA, IA2A, IAA and ZnT8-A antibodies) [37]. Nevertheless, the prevalence of SLE and autoimmune gestational diabetes, and the relationship between them, needs further research.

7.1 Lupus flare

During lupus pregnancies, there is an increased risk of maternal and fetal morbidity and mortality, but a stable disease prior to conception can act as predictor of a good outcome [38]. The onset of new symptoms or signs as arthritis, discoid or subacute cutaneous lupus lesions, oral ulcers, vasculitis, polyserositis, lymphadenopathy, positive direct Coombs, myocarditis, pneumonitis, proteinuria, leucopenia, thrombocytopenia, complement consumption or raised anti-DNA antibody expression must arise the suspicion about an ongoing lupus flare [12, 38].

During a healthy pregnancy, complement levels are usually raised, as it acts as acute phase reactant [31]. So, normal or lower range of complement suggests serum consumption due inflammatory process [38]. The coexistence of hypocomplementemia and high SLE activity usually predicts a poor pregnancy outcome. Proteinuria and leukopenia are also associated to a worse prognosis [31, 38].

Recently, the PROMISSE (Predictors of Pregnancy Outcome: Biomarkers in Antiphospholipid Antibody Syndrome and Systemic Lupus Erythematosus) study revealed that up to 20.8% lupus pregnancies experience mild to moderate flares but only 6.25% have severe ones [39]. Patients at risk were the ones with younger age, low C4 and higher physician global assessment at baseline as independent risk factors for having at least one flare during pregnancy. This study is remarkable and unique in that it has a multicenter, multiethnic and multiracial sample included. Hence, non-white race was also identified as a risk factor for lupus flare. According to the authors, there were no medications associated with flare, including hydroxychloroquine, in contrast to other studies.

SLE patients with central nervous system (CNS) involvement during pregnancy have higher risk for maternal and fetal complications and poor prognosis [40]. Preterm birth incidence can be 60% higher than in other lupus pregnancies and extreme prematurity can reach 40% of the newborns. CNS lupus pregnancies have higher risk for complications, whether neurological symptoms are present or not.

In contrast, in cutaneous lupus erythematosus the pregnancy outcomes are comparable to those of healthy populations [41].

As mentioned on Section 5.1, lupus patients can also have APS. Although rare, catastrophic APS (CAPS) can occur in up to 1% of patients and mortality reaches 50% [31].

7.2 Pre-eclampsia and lupus nephritis

Lupus nephritis (LN) is severe and independent risk factor for both maternal and fetal outcomes. It is related to preterm birth, hypertension and pre-eclampsia [42]. Pre-eclampsia have an increased risk in SLE pregnancy and can appear in up to 25% of SLE patients [31, 33]. Active LN at the time of conception has been pointed as the major risk factor for pre-eclampsia in SLE pregnancies [43]. LN activates in 4–30% of patients; those who had previous recurrence of LN are at a higher risk 20–30% [44].

The definition of pre-eclampsia by the International Society for the Study of Hypertension in Pregnancy Society (ISSHP) has recently been considered as being more sensitive than the definition made by the American College of Obstetricians and Gynecologists [45]. Pre-eclampsia is defined by the ISSHP as gestational hypertension, accompanied by at least one of the following conditions, at/or after 20 weeks' of gestation:

1. Proteinuria

2. Other maternal organ dysfunction, such as:

   a. Acute kidney injury (creatinine greater than 1 mg/dL)

   b. Liver involvement (alanine aminotransferase (ALT) or aspartate aminotransferase (AST) greater than 40 IU/L)

   c. Neurologic complications (eclampsia, altered mental status, blindness, stroke, clonus, severe headaches, persistent visual scotoma)

   d. Hematological complications (thrombocytopenia less than 150000/μL, disseminated intravascular coagulation, hemolysis)

3. Uteroplacental dysfunction – including fetal growth restriction, abnormal umbilical artery Doppler wave form analysis or stillbirth [46].

Therefore, after 20 weeks of gestation, the distinction between a lupus flare and pre-eclampsia can represent a diagnostic dilemma, since both can have similar characteristics – increased proteinuria, hypertension, thrombocytopenia, kidney dysfunction and generalized symptoms [31]. A thorough clinical history and biochemical investigation are always required. In a normal pregnancy, the complement is expected to be normal or high, since it acts as an acute phase reactant. If a normal or decreased range is detected, immune complexes are probably being formed and a lupus flare is ongoing. An increase of anti-DNA antibody levels is also related to lupus activity [31]. The onset of unexpected significant proteinuria should raise suspicion, especially if it occurs in the first trimester or part of the second trimester. In these cases, a proper clinical and laboratory approach is mandatory. In discordant results, renal biopsy can be considered. However, if aPL are present, the risk of thromboembolism should prompt to anticoagulation treatment, which would, in turn, raise the risk of major bleeding after biopsy. Other procoagulant factor include pregnancy itself, nephropathy, and SLE activity, so the need to a biopsy must be carefully outweighed [31].

If a patient develops only pre-eclampsia, it is not expected to find hematuria, urinary casts, complement consumption or increased anti-DNA antibodies [31]. On the other hand, LN can also induce pre-eclampsia, so, once again, the distinction of these two entities can be problematic. The correct diagnosis must be accurate, as the treatment approach will be totally different: in pre-eclampsia, the delivery should be anticipated; in LN, immunosuppressive treatment should be immediately started.

HELLP (Hemolysis with elevated liver enzymes and thrombocytopenia) syndrome is the worst manifestation of pre-eclampsia [22]. It is usually associated with aPL, but evidence has shown that it consists of a complementopathy, either due to an inherited defect in a complement regulatory protein or an acquired autoantibody [47]. *In vitro* experiments, using serum from HELLP patients in modified Ham test, disclosed activation of the alternative pathway of complement cascade (C5b-9). This dysregulation of complement system would be similar to that occurring in hemolytic uremic syndrome.

Although pre-eclampsia and LN exhibit different clinical manifestations, clear discrimination in the set of a new-onset SLE during pregnancy can be challenging – see **Table 2**. Soluble fms-like tyrosine kinase 1 (sFlt-1)/placental growth factor (PIGF) ratio can be useful in discriminating these two entities: women with SLE and APS who develop pre-eclampsia have a significantly higher sFlt-1/PIGF ratio compared with women with SLE and APS, but without pre-eclampsia [31, 48]. These variances increase during pregnancy.

7.3 Impact on fetal development and monitoring of fetal development during lupus pregnancy

As mentioned above, fetal risks of lupus pregnancy include pregnancy loss, preterm birth, premature rupture of membranes and FGR. Preterm birth is more frequent than pregnancy loss, and even if its relation to pre-eclampsia and disease activity is established, a causative factor may not be identified [22]. Other fetal complications associated with SLE include infants small for gestational age and infants with low birth weight [33]. Neonatal intensive care unit admissions are also more prevalent in these newborns.

Zhan Z et al., in a retrospective study identified that the best method to monitor adverse pregnancy complications during third trimester of pregnancy is by doing an umbilical artery Doppler. Nevertheless, the umbilical artery Doppler can be initiated in the second trimester in monitoring for neonatal heart block for possible earlier intervetion [49]. The use of hydroxychloroquine (HCQ) is associated with

Clinical measure	Preeclampsia	Lupus nephritis
Hypertension	After 20 weeks gestation	Any time during pregnancy
Urine active sediment	Rare	Common
Onset of proteinuria	Abrupt, after 20 weeks	Abrupt or gradual, anytime
Creatinine	Normal to raised	Normal to raised
Uric acid	Raised	Normal
C3 and C4	Usually normal	Usually low or decreasing
Complement products	Normal-low	Rising titres
Anti-DNA	Absent or unchanged	Normal to increased
Lupus activity	No	Yes
24 hour Urine calcium	<195 mg/day	>195 mg/day
Thrombocytopenia	Yes (HELLP)	20% of SLE
Other organ involvement	Occasionally CNS or HELLP	Evidence of active nonrenal SLE
Liver function test	May be elevated (HELLP)	Usually normal
Kidney biopsy	Glomeruloendotheliosis	SLE nephritis
sFlt-1/PIG ratio	Higher	Normal
Response to steroids	No	Yes

Abbreviations: HELLP - hemolysis, elevated liver enzymes, low platelets; SLE – systemic lupus erythematosus; sFlt-1 – soluble fms-like tyrosine kinase; PIGF – placental growth factor.

Table 2.
Differentiation of preeclampsia from lupus nephritis flare in pregnancy.

a lower incidence of FGR the risk of preterm delivery, whether spontaneous or induced, in lupus pregnancy [50, 51]. As prematurity decreases, there will also be a reduced risk of neonate complications, as respiratory distress syndrome, intraventicular hemorrhage, sepsis, hypoglycemia, jaundice requiring phototherapy, enterocolitis, among others [50]. Among the different studies done so far, it should be noted that children with in utero exposure to HCQ did not developed visual, auditory, developmental or growth abnormalities.

7.4 Delivery

The objective in a pregnant lupus patient would be a vaginal spontaneous delivery at term, data reveals that these women have a high prevalence of cesarean section. This procedure should be restricted to obstetric indications, once it represents an additional risk factor for venous thromboembolism, hemorrhage, infection and repercussion in future pregnancies. During labor, women exposed to long-term oral steroids may need intravenous hydrocortisone to overcome the physiologic stress of labor and delivery. Prophylactic or therapeutic anticoagulation should be interrupted as spontaneous delivery starts or, if induced labor or cesarean section is scheduled, it should be discontinued 12 or 24 hours before. Epidural or spinal anesthesia can be safely administrated until 12 hours after the last dose of anticoagulant.

Postpartum care must focus on a possible lupus flare or coexisting pre-eclampsia [31]. Women who underwent anticoagulation should continue it for at least 6 weeks after delivery in a prophylactic dose. Safe contraception should be offered and progestogens can be an appropriate option.

8. Treatment & prevention of complications during pregnancy

Therapeutic management in SLE patients is one of the most important aspects when planning a pregnancy. The main goal is to assure the most effective treatment to maintain disease remission, while keeping the ability to treat disease flares and guaranteeing maximum safety for the fetus. As mention on Section 3, disease activity should be under control (3 to 6 months) prior to pregnancy.

In order to decrease maternal and fetal complications, the the European League Against Rheumatism (EULAR) and the American College of Rheumatology (ACR) [20, 52] developed general recommendations describing which drugs are safe during pregnancy and which ones should be avoided. Also, the Unites States Food and Drug Administration (FDA) has changed the way of labelling medication safety during pregnancy and lactation. Previously, it was based on letters, which classified drugs from A to D, according to its increased risk for the fetus. Drugs classified as had not enough evidence or information available. Nowadays, this classification reflects more the quantity and quality of the data known for each drug. For practical proposes, the current drug options available to treat SLE pregnancy has been divided into 4 main categories:

8.1 Drugs recommended during SLE pregnancy

8.1.1 Hydroxychloroquine

Hydroxychloroquine (HCQ) is an antimalarial agent used for its immunomodulatory effects. Although HCQ crosses the placenta, it does not seem to have toxic effects on the fetus [53]. On the contrary, this drug is recommended to all women with SLE, whether they are pregnant or not, as it decreases the risk of flares, reduces the risk of pre-eclampsia and preterm birth [54]. Various studies have also shown positive effects of HCQ in pregnant women with APS (higher birth rates and fewer pregnancy complications) versus untreated patients, concluding that SLE pregnant women that have aPL, also known as "aPL carriers" also benefit from HCQ. Furthermore, some studies suggest that HCQ decreases the occurrence of CHB and cutaneous involvement in neonatal lupus, in fetuses whose mothers are carriers of anti-Ro/SSA and anti-La/SSB antibodies [55].

8.1.2 Low-dose acetylsalicylic acid

Low dose acetylsalicylic acid, as known as, "low dose aspirin" (LDA) is recommended in all women with SLE during pregnancy, it should be started during pre-conception period in case of a planned pregnancy and no later than 16 weeks. LDA (75-150 mg/day) has proved to reduce the risk of pre-eclampsia and its complications, regardless the presence of aPLs [56].

8.2 Drugs with a safe profile during pregnancy

The following drugs have an acceptable safety profile, but should be used selectively, if needed, to control SLE manifestations during pregnancy.

8.2.1 Non-steroidal anti-inflammatory drugs

Non-steroidal anti-inflammatory drugs (NSAIDs) are commonly used to control symptoms in patients with rheumatic diseases. However, these drugs should be prudently used during pre-conception period and during pregnancy, as they can provoke oligohydramnios, due to reduced fetal glomerular filtration rate. In case of absolute necessity, amniotic fluid monitoring is necessary [57].

Discordant findings from large retrospective studies have shown an increased risk of miscarriage in the first trimester with the use of NSAIDs [52]. These drugs should be avoided after 32 weeks of gestation, because of the risk of premature closure of the *ductus arteriosus,* with the exception of aspirin. Indomethacin and ibuprofen appear to have much stronger ductal effects than LDA [57].

Some studies suggest that high doses of aspirin may increase the risk of fetal or neonatal bleeding or bruising in the 3rd trimester. However, these data is not robust enough to warrant conclusions. The use of selective cyclooxygenase (COX)-2 inhibitors is not recommended in pregnancy, due to the lack of safety data [52, 58].

8.2.2 Glucocorticoids

Glucocorticoids (GC) have a remarkable path in the treatment of autoimmune diseases, such as SLE. Yet, its chronic use is associated with multiple side-effects and organ damage [59]. Prednisone and prednisolone are glucocorticoids recommended during pregnancy due to its pharmacokinetics and its shorter duration of action, since they are metabolized by placental enzymes the fetus is basically unexposed. The recommended daily dose should be $\leq$7.5 mg of prednisone. Doses superior to 10 mg/day are associated with preterm delivery, premature rupture of membranes and FGR. Higher doses should be reserved for organ-threatening situations, when the benefits outweigh the risks [60]. For hypothalamic–pituitary–adrenal axis suppression, for example, we use doses superior to 5 mg/day for at least 3 weeks, after the first trimester, so that labor and delivery can be managed accordingly.

Methylprednisolone has similar rates of placental transfer to prednisone so it is expected to be safe and compatible with pregnancy [20].

8.2.3 Azathioprine (AZA)

Azathioprine is especially used in SLE patients with hematological manifestations, but it can also be used in LN, as a maintenance drug [60]. This drug is compatible with pregnancy, since fetal liver lacks the enzyme to convert AZA to its active form [61]. Therefore, AZA is considered a safe drug, but doses should not exceed 2 mg/Kg/day.

8.2.4 Intravenous immunoglobulin

Intravenous immunoglobulin (IVIG) is an immunomodulator that regulates the inflammatory processes through anti-idiotype mechanisms. Although it crosses the placenta after the 2nd trimester and in a more significant way after the 3rd trimester, no fetal malformations have been reported. Hence, it is considered a drug compatible with pregnancy [62].

8.2.5 Cyclosporine and tacrolimus

Both cyclosporine (CSA) and tacrolimus are calcineurin inhibitors used as maintenance drugs and steroid-sparing agents, in patients with moderate to severe SLE [60]. CSA is considered safe in pregnancy, but blood pressure and renal function should be closely monitored [20]. It is recommended that CSA and tacrolimus should only be used when maternal benefit outweighs fetal risk, and preferably at minimum doses [63].

8.2.6 Antihypertensive medications

Metildopa, labetalol and hydralazine are frequently used during pregnancy with efficacy and no harm. Nifedipine is also compatible at doses up to 60 mg/day. By contrast, angiotensin-converting enzyme (ACE) inhibitors and angiotensin II receptor blockers are contraindicated throughout gestation and should be stopped as soon as possible, once pregnancy is confirmed. Diuretics can be used with caution and should be used as a last resource to control a severe and refractory hypertension, in an emergency setting and for a short period of time [20].

8.3 Drugs to be used with caution during pregnancy

8.3.1 Biologic agents

There is no sufficient data regarding biologic agents during pregnancy, so their use cannot be encouraged. Rituximab (RTX) is a B-cell depleting chimeric monoclonal antibody and is recommended to be stopped 6 months before conception. However, it has not been shown to be teratogenic [60, 64].

Belimumab (BEL) is BAFF inhibitor human monoclonal antibody and there is no sufficient data to recommend it during pregnancy. Until 12th week, IgG does not across placenta in significant amounts; so, accidental exposure to RTX or BEL during the first trimester is unlikely to be harmful. On the other hand, second/third trimester exposure will be associated with neonatal B-cell depletion [65].

8.4 Drugs contraindicated during pregnancy

8.4.1 Cyclophosphamide (CYC)

Cyclophosphamide (CYC) is an alkylating drug used in SLE, to treat severe organ or life-threatening manifestations [60]. Due to its teratogenic effects, its use in pregnancy is contraindicated, especially during the first trimester, when the fetus is more susceptible to congenital malformations. Nevertheless, it can be considered in exceptional circumstances, when mother faces an organ- or life-threatening disease complication. Embryotoxicity varies according to the stage of gestation. The use of this drug in fertile women should always be carefully evaluated and counseling about fertility preservation strategies should be advised prior to its use [66].

8.4.2 Mycophenolate mofetil

Mycophenolate mofetil (MMF) is an inhibitor of purine biosynthesis, commonly used in LN, as both in induction and maintenance therapy, and is also used in severe to refractory non-renal manifestations, with the exception of neuropsychiatric lupus [60]. Due to its teratogenic effects, its use in pregnancy is contraindicated. MMF exposure can cause lip and cleft palate, abnormalities of distal limbs and malformations of multiple internal organs, such as heart, esophagus and kidneys [67]. For these reasons, it should be avoided. Alternative options are azathioprine, tacrolimus or low dose of glucocorticoids, which can be used to control disease activity. They should be started, ideally, 6 months prior conception.

8.4.3 Methotrexate

Methotrexate (MTX) is a folate antagonist – it inhibits the enzyme dihydrofolate reductase which impairs purine and pyrimidine synthesis. It is contraindicated during pregnancy, due to its teratogenic effects. MTX exposure *in utero* can induce multiple congenital abnormalities, such as cleft palate, hydrocephalus, anencephaly and meningoencephalocele, delayed ossification and multiple facial deformities. It is strongly advised contraceptive use in patients taking MTX. This medication should be discontinued 3 months before attempting to conceive. If a woman is being treated with a low dose of MTX within 3 months prior to conception, or an accidental pregnancy occurs, the drug should be stopped immediately and the mother should continue to take folate supplementation (5 mg daily) throughout pregnancy. In the last case, a careful evaluation of fetal risk at an experienced center must take place [67].

8.4.4 Leflunomide

Leflunomide (LEF) is another drug that, although it may not be teratogenic, it is strongly advised to be avoided during pregnancy [68, 69]. It's an antimetabolite that inhibits dihydroorotate dehydrogenase, the catalyst enzyme responsible for the limiting step in pyrimidine biosynthesis. Despite its short half-life (approximately 15 days), its major metabolite follows a long path through enterohepatic circulation remaining detectable for more than 2 years. It is essential to complete its washout until undetectable levels before switching to alternative medication compatible with pregnancy and trying to conceive. For accelerate elimination of this drug, for example if an accidental pregnancy occurs, it is used cholestyramine (8 g orally, 3 times a day, for 11 days).

8.5 Management of maternal antiphospholipid syndrome

APL carriers or APS pregnancy represent a great challenge and require an additional monitoring and therapy to prevent maternal and/or fetal complications. Below is the clinical management according to the different clinical situations: [23, 52]

8.5.1 Asymptomatic aPL-positive patients "aPL carriers"

In SLE *aPL carriers* prophylaxis with LDA daily, is recommended during pregnancy. Combination therapy with prophylactic-dose heparin and LDA, even for those pregnant with triple-positive aPL or high LAC concentration, is not recommended [23, 52]. These women should be treated with prophylactic-dose low molecular weight heparin (LMWH) until, at least, 6 weeks after delivery.

8.5.2 Obstetric APS

In SLE women with history of obstetric complications prophylactic or therapeutic-dose heparin (usually LMWH) and LDA during gestation is recommended. Prophylactic or therapeutic-dose LMWH should continue until 6 weeks after delivery [23, 52].

8.5.3 Thrombotic APS

Women with previous thrombosis have a high risk of recurrent thrombotic event during pregnancy. Therefore, as soon as pregnancy is confirmed, vitamin K antagonists should be stopped, due to the fetotoxicity, and should be switched to therapeutic LMWH and LDA). LMWH and LDA should be stopped before delivery. Women with thrombotic APS are at very high risk of recurrent venous thromboembolism during post-partum. Therapeutic LMWH dose is recommended. Other possible option is to return to warfarin, which is safe during breastfeeding [23].

8.5.4 Refractory obstetric APS

Refractory Obstetric APS is a delicate and challenging situation, as there is no response to standard therapy. Some alternatives can be tried such as increased-dose of heparin (LMWH), low-dose prednisone (10 mg/day in the 1st trimester), IVIG, plasmapheresis, HCQ (5-6 mg/Kg/day). In 25% of obstetric APS, despite treatment, pregnancy loss can occur [23].

8.6 Management of SLE treatment and APS/aPLs positive patients in breastfeeding

Breastfeeding should be encouraged for all women and SLE patients are not an exception. However, some medications are transferred into the breast milk and can be harmful for the infant. Additionally, premature or ill infants are more susceptible to some medication's exposure [63, 69].

8.6.1 Drugs that are compatible with breastfeeding

Hydroxychloroquine is transferred to human breast milk, but only in an insignificant amount, about 2%, which is considered safe. Glucocorticoids, as prednisone or methylprednisolone, are considered compatible with breastfeeding, since they are excreted in the breast milk in very low quantities. It is accepted by the American Academy of Pediatrics and the British Society of Rheumatologists. Lactation is recommended to be avoided in the first 4 hours after ingestion of ≥20 mg of prednisone, as the peak concentration in breast milk is achieved 2 hours after maternal ingestion [63, 64].

Azathioprine, cyclosporine and tacrolimus, IVIG, heparin and warfarin are compatible with nursing, since the evidence shows that the excretion in breast milk is very low [63, 64].

Antihypertensive medications are commonly used, though evidence about the use of ACEIs and breastfeeding are lacking. Some data point out that captopril and/or enalapril seems to be selectively barred from blood to breast milk, so it is unlikely to cause adverse effects in nursing newborns. Nifedipine is considered safe during lactation [63, 70].

8.6.2 Drugs that are not compatible or should be avoided when breastfeeding

NSAIDs are not recommended, since there is not enough information about the safety of these drugs. Ibuprofen is the preferred drug, but only because it appears to be excreted in very small amounts in breast milk. Once more, LDA seems to be the exception, but there is no robust data about LDA and nursing.

Methotrexate is excreted in low concentrations into breast milk, but it can accumulate in neonatal tissues, so guidelines strongly advise to avoid MTX in breastfeeding mothers.

There is no sufficient data on the transmission of mycophenolate mofetil, leflunomide, RTX, BEL and in cyclophosphamide into breast milk, so these drugs should be avoided during lactation [58, 63, 70].

9. Postpartum and neonate complications

Maternal and fetal complications after pregnancy can result not only from SLE (disease), but also from other factors frequently associated with SLE. Maternal flares can occur in any trimester of pregnancy or after delivery, but it seems to be more prevalent in the 3rd trimester and until one year after delivery. Thus, the importance of maternal (and newborn) monitoring in the first year after delivery is of extreme importance [71–74].

9.1 Maternal complications of postpartum SLE

In a healthy SLE pregnancy, the woman should be offered the chance to a spontaneous labor, at term, with vaginal delivery [75]. Maternal medication may need a special adjustment for labor: intravenous hydrocortisone to overcome its physiological stress, discontinuation of LMWH, for which the timing will condition regional anesthesia.

As mentioned, SLE is associated with a higher incidence of maternal complications, both during pregnancy and in the postpartum period. Pregnant women with SLE are more likely to have a cesarean section (unplanned), high blood pressure, pre-eclampsia, spontaneous abortion, thromboembolic events, and infections [20]. In patients under corticosteroids at immunosuppressive dose (≥1 mg/Kg), prophylactic antibiotics is recommended, due to the risk of infections and sepsis [75].

HELLP syndrome (characterized by hemolysis, elevated liver enzymes and a low platelet count in the context of pregnancy) can, by definition, occur in the postpartum period. This occurs in one third of the cases, being more prevalent in women with severe pre-eclampsia [43]. Catastrophic antiphospholipid syndrome (CAPS), characterized by acute thrombotic micro-angiopathy, was also recorded in the postpartum period [76]. These syndromes are more frequent in patients with SLE, thus increasing the risk of complications in this population.

The postpartum period demands a rigorous monitoring for maternal complications, as SLE flare [75]. Although no increased risk of lupus flares between 2 and 6 months postpartum, compared to during pregnancy, was found, which rate is about 24%, flares can reach almost every patient in the first 6 months after delivery [39]. The treatment for these situations is similar for non-pregnant SLE patients, but the risks of breastfeeding under aggressive therapy should be outweighed. LMHW should be continued for 6 weeks after delivery, due to the increased risk of venous thromboembolism (VTE) during puerperium. Contraception should be encouraged, but estrogen-containing pills must not be used by women with aPL antibodies or APS, moderate to severe SLE and other conditions, as previous VTE, hypertension, obesity or smoking.

9.2 Newborn complications of SLE

In general, SLE in pregnancy is associated with a higher incidence of stillbirths, a greater occurrence of great premature babies, with a greater number of newborns admitted to neonatal intensive care units, an APGAR score below 7 within 1 and 5 minutes and a significantly higher number of birth defects [33, 77, 78].

Neonatal SLE (0 to 27 days after delivery) is an autoimmune disease that results from passive transfer of autoantibodies from a mother with SLE to the fetus, resulting in fetal and neo-natal disease. It occurs in about 3.5–8% of theses pregnancies and is associated with the presence of maternal anti-Ro/SSA and anti-La/SSB autoantibodies [20, 79]. Main manifestations involve cutaneous and cardiac systems, but it can affect and cause other organ dysfunctions (including thrombocytopenia, hepatitis, and myocarditis) [71]. The presence of anti-Ro/SSA antibodies may be associated with clinical manifestations, but does not appear to have a negative impact on other SLE-related events during pregnancy [80].

The most frequent manifestation of SLE in the neonate, with a prevalence of 10 to 20%, is a transient cutaneous rash with annular or elliptical erythematous plaques, which develops in the weeks following delivery [80]. It involves predominantly the face and scalp, is generally photosensitive and resolves spontaneously in the first 6 to 8 months of life, which coincides with the clearance of maternal autoantibodies from the circulation [71].

The most serious complication of neonatal SLE is a CHB, which can be diagnosed in-utero, on the date of birth or in the neonatal period. This occurs in about 2% of the fetuses of women with anti-Ro/SSA antibodies with a recurrence rate of 20% in the following pregnancies [76, 81, 82]. CHB can be of any degree and can be accompanied by extra-nodal disease, with valve involvement, endocardial (endocardial fibroelastosis) or structural changes, including dilated cardiomyopathy. About 60% of CHB babies will require a pacemaker; 10% of those will develop cardiomyopathy after birth [12]. The 10-year mortality rate ranges 20–35%. The use of HCQ during pregnancy seems to reduce in 65% the risk of cardiac manifestations of neonatal lupus in women with anti-Ro/SSA and anti-La/SSB autoantibodies [83, 84]. Despite immunoglobulin can reduce transplacental transfer of anti-Ro/SSA antibodies, a clinical trial failed to prove its efficacy [22].

Management of SLE pregnancy includes serial fetal echocardiography surveillance between 16 and 28 weeks of gestation [22]. If CHB is detected, it is usually no longer reversible. However, corticosteroids that are transplacental, as dexamethasone, can be administrated in order to reduce the resultant cardiomyopathy.

Prognostic factors related to poor outcomes of neonatal CHB include: detection of CHB at gestational age < 20 weeks, ventricular rate < 50 bpm, fetal hydrops, carditis, changes in fetal echocardiogram, endocardial fibroelastosis, impaired left ventricular function, and a maternal diagnosis of SLE or Sjögren's syndrome [12].

10. Conclusion

The improvement in disease management and pregnancy monitoring have resulted in a significant decrease in maternal and fetal complications in the last few decades. This has been mainly contributed by 3 pillars: 1) new technologies – which have permitted a better understanding of the immunopathogenesis of the disease, enabling substantial data on SLE patients and focusing on the area of genetics, such as genetic predisposition, epigenetics contribution and how these contribute in developing irreversible loss of immunologic self-tolerance; 2) access to healthcare – has permitted SLE patients to better hospital care through the course of their disease; and most importantly: 3) multidisciplinary management – this is essential to achieve successful maternal and fetal outcomes. This is made by a multidisciplinary team of experienced and dedicated physicians that define a strategic plan, such as preconception counseling, pregnancy planning and increased availability of safe drugs in pregnancy and puerperium, to improve both maternal and fetal outcomes. It is crucial to make the correct choice of therapy for women with SLE preconceptionally, during pregnancy and lactation. Medications must be reviewed and adjusted to minimize the effect on the fetus, while maintaining the disease under control.

In this way, even if SLE keeps being a severe risk factor for pregnancy, a healthy outcome for both mother and child has become a more frequent reality.

Author details

Melissa Fernandes[1*], Vera Bernardino[1,2], Anna Taulaigo[1], Jorge Fernandes[1], Ana Lladó[1,2] and Fátima Serrano[2,3]

1 Internal Medicine Department, Hospital Curry Cabral, Centro Hospitalar Universitário Lisboa Central, Lisbon, Portugal

2 Nova Medical School, Universidade Nova de Lisboa, Lisbon, Portugal

3 Obstetric Department, Maternidade Alfredo da Costa, Centro Hospitalar Universitário Lisboa Central, Lisbon, Portugal

*Address all correspondence to: melissa.a.fernandes@gmail.com

References

[1] Zen M, Iaccarino L, Gatto M, et al. Prolonged remission in Caucasian patients with SLE: prevalence and outcomes. Ann Rheum Dis. 2015; 74: 2117-22.

[2] Baglio V, Gharbiya M, Balacco-Gabrieli C, et al. Choroidopathy in patients with systemic lupus erythematosus with or without nephropathy. J Nephrol. 2011; 24: 522-9.

[3] Nguyen QD, Uy HS, Akpek EK, et al. Choroidopathy of systemic lupus erythematosus. Lupus. 2000; 9: 288-98.

[4] Rees F, Doherty M, Grainge MJ, Lanyon P, Zhang W. The worldwide incidence and prevalence of systemic lupus erythematosus: a systematic review of epidemiological studies. Rheumatology (Oxford). 2017 Nov 1;56(11):1945-1961.

[5] Rodrigues Senna E, De Barros ALP, Silva EO et al. Prevalence of rheumatic diseases in Brazil: a study using the COPCORD approach. J Rheumatol 2004;31 (Suppl 3):5947.

[6] Chakravarty EF, Bush TM, Manzi S, Clarke AE, Ward MM. Prevalence of adult systemic lupus erythematosus in California and Pennsylvania in 2000: estimates obtained using hospitalization data. Arthritis Rheum. 2007 Jun;56(6):2092-4.

[7] Tosounidou S, Bertsias G, Gordon C, Boumpas DT. (2015). Chapter 20 – Systemic Lupus Erythematosus: Pathogenesis and Clinical Features. Eular Textbook on Rheumatic Diseases. Saudi Med J. 2015;36(12):1503.

[8] Aranow C, Diamond B, Mackay M. Chapter 51 - Systemic Lupus Erythematosus, Editor(s): Robert R. Rich, Thomas A. Fleisher, William T. Shearer, Harry W. Schroeder, Anthony J. Frew, Cornelia M. Weyand, Clinical Immunology (Fifth Edition), Elsevier, 2019:685-704.

[9] Goulielmos GN, Zervou MI, Vazgiourakis VM, et al. The genetics and molecular pathogenesis of systemic lupus erythematosus (SLE) in populations of different ancestry. Gene. 2018 Aug 20;668:59-72.

[10] Ostensen M, Clowse M, "Pathogenesis of pregnancy complications in systemic lupus erythematosus," Current Opinion in Rheumatology, vol. 25, no. 5, pp. 591-596, 2013.

[11] Förger, F., Villiger, P.M. Immunological adaptations in pregnancy that modulate rheumatoid arthritis disease activity. Nat Rev Rheumatol 16, 113-122 (2020).

[12] Jesus GR, Pinto CM, Jesus NR, et al. "Understanding and Managing Pregnancy in Patients with Lupus,"Autoimmune Diseases, Vol 2015

[13] Gluhovschi C, Gluhovschi G, Petrica L, et al. Pregnancy Associated with Systemic Lupus Erythmatosus: Immune Tolerance in Pregnancy and its Deficiency in Systemic Lupus Erythematosus – An Immunological Dilemma. Journal of Immunology Research, vol. 2015.

[14] J. Ernerudh, G. Berg, and J. Mjösberg, "Regulatory T helper cells in pregnancy and their roles in systemic versus local immune tolerance," *The American Journal of Reproductive Immunology*, vol. 66, supplement 1, pp. 31-43, 2011.

[15] Talaat RM, Mohamed SF, Bassyouni IH, Raouf AA. Th1/Th2/Th17/Treg cytokine imbalance in systemic lupus erythematosus (SLE) patients: Correlation with disease activity. Cytokine. 2015 Apr;72(2):146-53.

[16] Dolff S, Bijl M, Huitema MG, Limburg PC, Kallenberg CG, Abdulahad WH.Clin Immunol. 2011 Nov;141(2):197-204.

[17] Tavakolpour S, Rahimzadeh G. New Insights into the Management of Patients with Autoimmune Diseases or Inflammatory Disorders During Pregnancy. Scand J Immunol. 2016 Sep;84(3):146-9.

[18] Walker SE. Estrogen and autoimmune disease. Clin Rev Allergy Immunol. 2011 Feb;40(1):60-5.

[19] Torricelli M, Bellisai F, Novembri R, et al., "High levels of maternal serum IL-17 and activin A in pregnant women affected by systemic lupus erythematosus," *The American Journal of Reproductive Immunology*, vol. 66, no. 2, pp. 84-89, 2011.

[20] Andreoli L, Bertsias GK, Agmon-Levin N, *et al.* EULAR recommendations for women's health and the management of family planning, assisted reproduction, pregnancy and menopause in patients with systemic lupus erythematosus and/ or antiphospholipid syndrome *Annals of the Rheumatic Diseases* 2017;**76:**476-485.

[21] Lateef A, Petri M. Managing lupus patients during pregnancy. Best Pract Res Clin Rheumatol. 2013 Jun;27(3): 435-47.

[22] Petri M. Pregnancy and Systemic Lupus Erythematosus. Best Pract Res Clin Obstet Gynaecol. 2020 Apr;64: 24-30.

[23] Fernandes MA, Gerardi MC, Andreoli L, Tincani A. Management of maternal antiphospholipid syndrome. Clin Exp Rheumatol. 2020 Jan-Feb; 38(1):149-156.

[24] Andreoli L, Gerardi MC, Fernandes M, et al. Disease activity assessment of rheumatic diseases during pregnancy: a comprehensive review of indices used in clinical studies. Autoimmun Rev. 2019 Feb;18(2): 164-176.

[25] Nahal SK, Selmi C, Gershwin ME. Safety issues and recommendations for successful pregnancy outcome in systemic lupus erythematosus. J Autoimmun. 2018 Sep;93:16-23.

[26] De Carolis S, Moresi S, Rizzo F, Monteleone G, Tabacco S, Salvi S, Garufi C, Lanzone A. Autoimmunity in obstetrics and autoimmune diseases in pregnancy. Best Pract Res Clin Obstet Gynaecol. 2019 Oct;60:66-76.

[27] Fischer-Betz R, Specker C. Pregnancy in systemic lupus erythematosus and antiphospholipid syndrome. Best Pract Res Clin Rheumatol. 2017 Jun;31(3):397-414.

[28] Mowla K, Alwanian M, Bahadoram S et al. Lupus nephritis in pregnancy; a mini-review to current knowledge. J Renal Inj Prev. 2018;7(1):42-44.

[29] Datta S et al. Obstetric Anesthesia Handbook. Springer Science + Business Media, LLC 2006, 2010.

[30] Ouzounian J, Elkayam U. Physiologic Changes During Normal Pregnancy and Delivery. Cardiol Clin. 2012;30:317-329.

[31] Ordi-Ros J, Marce CS and Cortes-Hernandez J. Lupus Pregnancy: Risk Factors and Management. IntechOpen. 2019

[32] Sharma P, Singh A, Mahopatra TK, et al. Physical physiological and biochemical changes during pregnancy. Santosh University Journal of Health Sciences. 2018;4(2):58-62.

[33] He WR and Wei H. Maternal and fetal complications associated with lupus erythematosus – an update

meta-analysis of the most recent studies (2017-2019). Medicine. 2020;99:16.

[34] Moroni G and Ponticelli C. Pregnancy in women with systemic lupus erythematosus (SLE). European Journal of Medicine. 2016;32:7-12.

[35] Clowse MEB, Jamison M, Myers E, et al. A national study of the complications of lupus in pregnancy. Am J Obstet Gynecol 2008;199:127.e1-127.e6.

[36] Dong Y, Dai Z, Wang Z, et al. Risk of gestational diabetes mellitus in systemic lupus erythematosus pregnancy: a systematic review and meta-analysis. BMC Pregnancy and Childbirth. 2019;19:179.

[37] Cossu E, Incani M, Pani MG, et al. Presence of diabetes-specific autoimmunity in women with gestational diabetes mellitus (GDM) predicts impaired glucose regulation at follow-up. J Endocrinol Investig. 2018; 41:1061-8.

[38] Parastandechehr G, Faezi ST, Paragomi P et al. Can pregnancy induce relapse in systemic lupus erythematosus (SLE)?. Rheumatology Research Journal. 2016;1(1):27-32.

[39] Davis-Porada, J, Kim M, Guerra M, et al. Low frequency of flares during pregnancy and post-partum in stable lupus patients. Arthritis Research & Therapy. 2020;22:52.

[40] El-Sayed YY, Lu EJ, Genovese MC et al. Central nervous system lupus and pregnancy: 11-year experience at a single center. The Journal of Maternal-Fetal & Neonatal Medicine. 2002;12(2): 99-103.

[41] Hamed H, Ahmed S, Alzolibani A et al. Does cutaneous lupus erythematosus have more favorable pregnancy outcomes than systemic disease? A two-center study. Acta Obstetricia et Gynecologica Scandinavica. 2013;92:934-942.

[42] Moroni G and Ponticelli C. Important considerations in pregnant patients with lupus nephritis. Expert Review of Clinical Immunology. 2018;14:489-498.

[43] Stogan G, Baer AN. Flares of systemic lupus erythematosus during pregnancy and the puerperium: prevention, diagnosis and management. Expert review of clinical immunology. 2012;8(5):439-53.

[44] Clowse ME. Lupus activity in pregnancy. Rheuma Dis Clin North Am. 2007;33:237-52.

[45] Lai J, Syngelaki A, Nicolaides K, et al. Impact of new definitions of preeclampsia at term on identification of adverse maternal and perinatal outcomes. Am J of Obstet Gynecol. 2020 Nov 6;S0002-9378(20)31286-2. doi: 10.1016/j.ajog.2020.11.004.

[46] Brown MA, Magee LA, Kenny LC, et al. The hypertensive disorders of pregnancy: ISSHP classification, diagnosis & management recommendations for international practice. Pregnancy Hypertens. 2018;13:291-310.

[47] Vaught AJ, Gavriilaki E, Hueppchen N, et al. Direct evidence of complement activation in HELLP syndrome: a link to atypical hemolytic uremic syndrome. Exp Hematol. 2016;1;44(5):390-8.

[48] Hirashima C, Ogoyama M, Abe M, et al. Clinical usefulness of sérum levels of soluble fms-like tyrosine kinase 1/ placental growth factor ratio to rule out preeclampsia in women with new-onset lupus nephritis during pregnancy. CEN Case Reports. 2019;8:95-100.

[49] Zhan Z, Yang Y, Zhan Y et al. Fetal outcomes and associated factors of

adverse outcomes of pregnancy in southern Chinese women with systemic lupus erythematosus. PLoS One. 2017;12:e0176457.

[50] Leroux M, Desveaux C, Parcevaux M, et alt. Impact of hydroxychloroquine on preterm delivery and intrauterine growth restriction in pregnant women with systemic lupus erythematosus: a description cohort study. Lupus. 2015,0:1-8.

[51] Canti V, Scarrone M, De Lorenzo R et al. Low incidence of intrauterine restriction in pregnant patients with systemic lupus erythematosus taking hydroxychloroquine. Immunological Medicine. 2021.

[52] Sammaritano LR, Bermas BL, Chakravarty EE, et al. 2020 American College of Rheumatology Guidelines for the Management of Reprodutive Heath in Rheumatic and Musculoskeletal Diseases. Arthritis Rheumatol 2020; 72:529.

[53] Yang H, Liu H, Xu D, et al. Pregnancy-related systemic lupus erythematosus: clinical features, outcome and risk factores of disease flares – a case control study. PLoS One 2014; 9:e104375.

[54] Schrezenmeier E, Dörner T. Mechanisms of action of hydroxychloroquine and chloroquine: implications for rheumatology. Nat Rev Rheumatol. 2020;16:155-166.

[55] Barsalou J, Costedoat-Chalumeau N, Berhanu A, et al. Effect of in utero hydroxychloroquine exposure on the development of cutaneous neonatal lupus erythematosus. Ann Rheum Dis. 2018;77:1742-1749.

[56] LeFevre ML, U.S. Preventive Services Task Force. Low-dose aspirin use for prevention of morbidity and mortality from preeclampsia: U.S. Preventive Services Task Force recommendation statement. Ann Intern Med 2014; 161:819.

[57] Koren G, Florescu A, Costei AM, et al. Nonsteroidal antiinflammatory drugs during third trimester and the risk of premature closure of the ductus arteriosus: A meta-analysis. Ann Pharmacother. 2006;40:824-829.

[58] Flint J, Panchal S, Hurrell A, et al. BSR and BHPR guideline on prescribing drugs in pregnancy and breastfeeding — Part II : analgesics and other drugs used in rheumatology practice. Rheumatology (Oxford). 2016;1-31.

[59] Bruce IN, Urowitz M, van Vollenhoven R, et al. Long-term organ damage accrual and safety in patients with SLE treated with belimumab plus standard of care. Lupus. 2016;25: 699-709.

[60] Fanouriakis A, Kostopoulou M, Alunno A, et al. 2019 update of the EULAR recommendations for the management of systemic lupus erythematosus. Ann Rheum Dis. 2019;78:736-745.

[61] Andreoli L, Fredi M, Nalli C, et al. Pregnancy implications for systemic lupus erythematosus and the antiphospholipid syndrome. J Autoimmun. 2012;38.

[62] Porta S, Danza A, Arias Saavedra M, et al. Glucocorticoids in Systemic Lupus Erythematosus. Ten Questions and Some Issues. J Clin Med. 2020;9:2709.

[63] Flint J, Panchal S, Hurrell A, et al. BSR and BHPR guideline on prescribing drugs in pregnancy and breastfeeding- Part I: Standard and biologic disease modifying anti-rheumatic drugs and corticosteroids. Rheumatol (United Kingdom). 2016;55:1693-1697.

[64] Flint J, Panchal S, Hurrel A, et al. BSR and BHPR guideline on prescribing

drugs in pregnancy and breastfeeding – Part II: analgesics and other drugs used in Rheumatology practice. Rheumatology (Oxford). 2016;1699-1701.

[65] Turner-Stokes T, Lu TY, Ehrenstein MR, et al. The efficacy of repeated treatment with B-cell depletion therapy in systemic lupus erythematosus: an evaluation. Rheumatology (Oxford). 2011;50: 1401-1408.

[66] Navarra S V., Guzmán RM, Gallacher AE, et al. Efficacy and safety of belimumab in patients with active systemic lupus erythematosus: A randomised, placebo-controlled, phase 3 trial. Lancet. 2011;377:721-731.

[67] Vaux KK, Kahole NCO, Jones KL. Cyclophosphamide, Methotrexate, and Cytarabine Embropathy: Is Apoptosis the Common Pathway? Birth Defects Res Part A - Clin Mol Teratol. 2003;67:403-408.

[68] Cassina M, Johnson DL, Robinson LK, et al. Pregnancy outcome in women exposed to leflunomide before or during pregnancy. Arthritis Rheum 2012; 64:2085.

[69] Østensen M, Khamashta M, Lockshin M, et al. Anti-inflammatory and immunosuppressive drugs and reproduction. Arthritis Res Ther. 2006;8:209.

[70] Drugs and lactation database (LactMed) of the United Sates National Library of Medicine http://toxnet.nlm.nih.gov

[71] Baer AN, Witter FR, Petri M. Lupus and pregnancy. *Obstet Gynecol Surv*. 2011;66(10):639-653.

[72] Andreoli L, García-Fernández A, Chiara Gerardi M, Tincani A. The Course of Rheumatic Diseases During Pregnancy. *Isr Med Assoc J*. 2019;21(7):464-470.

[73] Ko HS, Ahn HY, Jang DG, et al. Pregnancy outcomes and appropriate timing of pregnancy in 183 pregnancies in Korean patients with SLE. *Int J Med Sci*. 2011;8(7):577-583.

[74] Götestam Skorpen C, Lydersen S, Gilboe IM, et al. Disease Activity During Pregnancy and the First Year Postpartum in Women With Systemic Lupus Erythematosus. *Arthritis Care Res (Hoboken)*. 2017;69(8):1201-1208.

[75] Pastore D, Costa ML, Parpinelli MA, Surita F. A Critical Review on Obstetric Follow-up of Women Affected by Systemic Lupus Erythematosus. Rev Bras Ginecol Obstet. 2018;40:209-2024.

[76] Buyon JP, Hiebert R, Copel J, et al. Autoimmune-associated congenital heart block: demographics, mortality, morbidity and recurrence rates obtained from a national neonatal lupus registry. *J Am Coll Cardiol*. 1998;31(7):1658-1666.

[77] Bundhun PK, Soogund MZ, Huang F. Impact of systemic lupus erythematosus on maternal and fetal outcomes following pregnancy: A meta-analysis of studies published between years 2001-2016. *J Autoimmun*. 2017;79:17-27.

[78] Yasmeen S, Wilkins EE, Field NT, Sheikh RA, Gilbert WM. Pregnancy outcomes in women with systemic lupus erythematosus. *J Matern Fetal Med*. 2001;10(2):91-96.

[79] Kwok LW, Tam LS, Zhu T, Leung YY, Li E. Predictors of maternal and fetal outcomes in pregnancies of patients with systemic lupus erythematosus. *Lupus*. 2011;20(8):829-836.

[80] Brucato A, Cimaz R, Caporali R, Ramoni V, Buyon J. Pregnancy outcomes in patients with autoimmune diseases and anti-Ro/SSA antibodies. *Clin Rev Allergy Immunol*. 2011;40(1):27-41.

[81] Gordon P, Khamashta MA, Rosenthal E, et al. Anti-52 kDa Ro, anti-60 kDa Ro, and anti-La antibody profiles in neonatal lupus. *J Rheumatol*. 2004;31(12):2480-2487.

[82] Izmirly PM, Rivera TL, Buyon JP. Neonatal lupus syndromes. *Rheum Dis Clin North Am*. 2007;33(2):267-vi.

[83] Izmirly PM, Kim MY, Llanos C, et al. Evaluation of the risk of anti-SSA/Ro-SSB/La antibody-associated cardiac manifestations of neonatal lupus in fetuses of mothers with systemic lupus erythematosus exposed to hydroxychloroquine. *Ann Rheum Dis*. 2010;69(10):1827-1830.

[84] Izmirly P, Saxena A, Buyon JP. Progress in the pathogenesis and treatment of cardiac manifestations of neonatal lupus. *Curr Opin Rheumatol*. 2017;29(5):467-472.

Section 5

Lupus: The Advent in Disease Targeted Therapy Current and Future Perspectives

Chapter 6

Novel Therapeutic Interventions in Systemic Lupus Erythematosus

Panagiotis Athanassiou, Lambros Athanassiou and Ifigenia Kostoglou-Athanassiou

Abstract

Systemic lupus erythematosus (SLE) is a systemic autoimmune disease. It is characterized by a variable clinical course ranging from mild to fatal disease. It can affect the kidneys. The aim of treatment in SLE is the prevention of flares and the prevention of accumulation of damage to the main organs affected as well as the prevention of drug side effects. The cornerstone of SLE treatment is hydroxychloroquine. Corticosteroids are used both as induction treatment in disease flares as well as in small doses as maintenance treatment. Immunosuppressants, such as azathioprine, methotrexate and mycophenolate mofetil are used as steroid sparing agents. Calcineurin inhibitors, namely tacrolimus and cyclosporin A may also be used as immunosuppressants and steroid sparing agents. Pulse methylprednisolone, along with mycophenolate mofetil and cyclophosphamide are used as induction treatment in lupus nephritis. Rituximab, an anti-CD20 biologic agent may be used in non-renal SLE. In patients insufficiently controlled with hydroxychloroquine, low dose prednisone and/or immunosuppressive agents, belimumab may be used with beneficial effects in non-renal disease and lupus nephritis.

Keywords: systemic lupus erythematosus, treatment, hydroxychloroquine, corticosteroids, mycophenolate mofetil, rituximab, belimumab

1. Introduction

Systemic lupus erythematosus (SLE) is a systemic autoimmune disease affecting many organ systems. It has a variable course, ranging from a mild course to severe fatal disease. It affects mainly women in the reproductive age. Women of African or Asian origin suffer frequently and present with more severe disease. The treatment of SLE is in the focus of scientific interest as new immune modulating agents have entered the management of the disease.

The therapeutic management of the disease depends mainly on antimalarial agents, namely hydroxychloroquine, corticosteroids, immunosuppressive agents and biologic drugs (**Figures 1** and **2**). The use of hydroxychloroquine is established in SLE. Similarly, the use of corticosteroids has been in the mainstream of lupus treatment for many years. Their use is hindered by their adverse effects, which may occur even with small doses. Immunosuppressive agents such as azathioprine and methotrexate have been used as steroid sparing agents. The use of mycophenolate mofetil (MMF) is also in the mainstream treatment of severe SLE cases or lupus nephritis. Rituximab, an antiCD20 antibody targeting B lymphocytes has also been

 IntechOpen

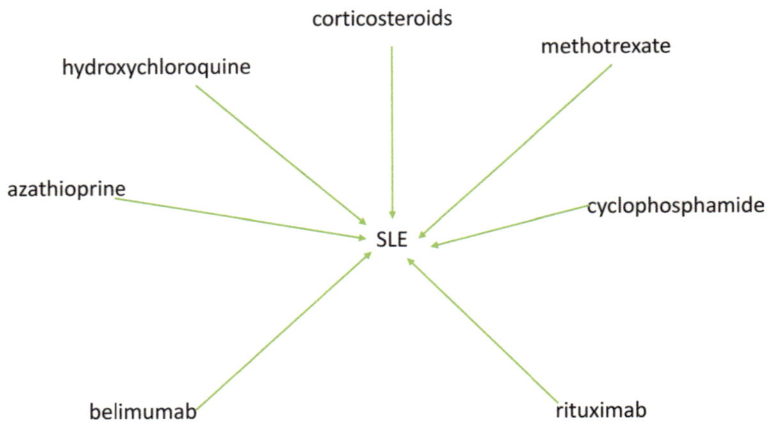

Figure 1.
Agents involved in systemic lupus erythematosus treatment.

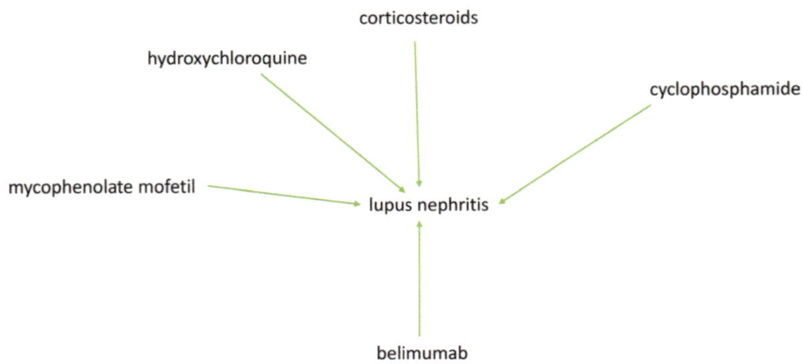

Figure 2.
Agents contributing to the treatment of lupus nephritis.

applied in the treatment of severe SLE cases. Recently, the use of belimumab has been introduced in the treatment of SLE and is indicated in patients with non-renal disease and renal disease not responsive to standard treatment. Although, recent advances in treatment have improved prognosis and life expectancy in lupus patients, much progress remains to be achieved. In the present chapter, the use of various treatment modalities for SLE will be discussed. Additionally, the use of supplementary drugs will be reviewed.

2. Systemic lupus erythematosus treatment

2.1 Antimalarials

Antimalarials have been used for many years in the treatment of rheumatic diseases [1, 2]. Historically, antimalarials had been observed to ameliorate rheumatic symptoms in soldiers taking these drugs during World War II for the prevention of malaria [3]. Clinical application of hydroxychloroquine and chloroquine in the treatment of rheumatic diseases has been widely reported. The use of hydroxychloroquine in the treatment of SLE has been well established [4, 5]. It has been used in both discoid lupus and SLE [6]. Chloroquine and hydroxychloroquine increase pH within intracellular vacuoles and modify processes such as protein degradation by acidic hydrolases in the lysosome, organization of macromolecules in the endosomes, and post-translation modification of proteins in the Golgi apparatus. The antirheumatic properties of antimalarials is a consequence of their interference with antigen processing in antigen-presenting cells. For the digestion of antigenic proteins and for the peptides to assemble with the chains of the MHC class II proteins it is necessary to have acidic cytoplasmic compartments. Antimalarials increase the pH thereby diminishing the formation of peptide-MHC protein complexes which are required to stimulate CD4+ T cells and down-regulating the immune response against autoantigenic peptides [7, 8]. It also blocks Toll-like receptors on dendritic cells [9]. A review of controlled trials on the clinical efficacy and safety of antimalarials showed that adequate evidence exist for these drugs, in particular hydroxychloroquine in preventing lupus flares, increasing long term survival of patients and lupus activity in pregnant women without proven teratogenicity [10]. Moderate evidence exists for the prevention of irreversible organ damage, prevention of bone destruction and prevention of thrombosis. Weaker evidence exists for the reduction in severe lupus activity, lipid levels and subclinical atherosclerosis [11]. Hydroxychloroquine has been shown to improve glucose metabolism [12]. The toxicity of antimalarials is mild, infrequent and it is usually reversible. When given attention to dosage hydroxychloroquine has a safer profile. Ruiz-Irastorza et al recommended that hydroxychloroquine should be given to all patients with lupus during the full course of the disease [13]. They have described hydroxychloroquine as being the cornerstone of lupus treatment [13]. There have been very few efforts on discontinuation of the drug due to its proven efficacy and the few and mild side effects. Hydroxychloroquine has multiple beneficial effects in SLE. It reduces lipid levels, thereby inhibiting atherosclerosis [14, 15]. Hydroxychloroquine has multiple effects on cholesterol metabolism, as it inhibits cholesterol biosynthesis, inihibits lysosomal hydrolysis of cholesteryl ester and stimulates the capacity of LDL receptor and the activity of HMG-CoA reductase [16]. Hydroxychloroquine protects lupus patients from thrombosis, as it has known antithrombotic action. It reduces red blood sludging, blood viscosity, platelet aggregation and protects the annexin V "shield" from disruption by antiphospholipid antibodies [17]. Additionally, it reduces glucose levels via multiple mechanisms [18].

2.2 Corticosteroids

Corticosteroids have been used at large bolus doses as induction treatment as well as at small doses as maintenance treatment in patients with SLE [19] (**Figure 1**). They reduce disease activity as well as disease burden accrual on different organ systems [20]. Corticosteroids have potent immunomodulatory properties [21]. They are known to modulate all aspects of immune response and have strong immunosuppressive and anti-inflammatory properties [22, 23]. Their effects on the immune system are known to be mediated mainly by their trans repression mode of action, namely by their ability to reduce the expression of inflammatory transcription factors [24]. As corticosteroids are characterized by many severe and less severe side effects such as propensity to infections [25, 26], blood glucose elevation [27] and osteoporosis [28], different immunomodulating agents have been applied in patients with SLE as corticosteroid sparing agents.

Methylprednisolone pulse therapy is used for the treatment of severe manifestations of SLE. Intravenous pulses of prednisolone rapidly immunosuppress patients with organ and/or life-threatening manifestations of SLE [29, 30]. The gold standard is 1 g/day for 3-5 days [31]. However, this treatment schedule may be associated with significant infectious complications and lower doses may be useful as well. In particular, it has been shown that a lower dose pulse methylprednisolone treatment schedule involving ≤1500 mg/3 days may have the same beneficial effects and fewer adverse effects, in particular severe infections [32]. An intensive treatment schedule of rituximab, cyclophosphamide and intravenous pulses of methylprednisolone has been applied with excellent results in patients with SLE and severe organ manifestations including nephritis [33]. Patients improved significantly and long-term immunosuppression other than prednisone 5 mg/day was avoided.

Corticosteroids in the form of prednisone daily as maintenance treatment for SLE patients has been applied for years. New data show that introducing lower initial doses of prednisone (<15 mg/day) and thereafter tapering to low doses of prednisone (5 mg/day or even lower) has been shown to be effective in SLE [34–36]. Mild flares can be managed with transient increases of prednisone up to 15 mg/day with rapid reduction. In moderate severe flares the use of pulse methylprednisolone 125 mg, 250 mg or 500 mg/day for three consecutive days is much more effective and less toxic than increasing oral prednisone to 0.5-1 mg/kg/day [32]. Rapid reduction from doses up to 30 mg/day prednisone should be performed to 5-2.5 mg/day within few weeks. Immunosuppressive therapy should be started early in severe forms of the disease and when prednisone cannot be reduced to 5 mg/day or less.

2.3 Immunosuppressants

2.3.1 Azathioprine

Azathioprine is a purine analogue. It inhibits DNA synthesis by acting on proliferating cells [37]. It acts on the DNA [38]. Azathioprine is metabolized to 6-mercaptopurine through reduction by glutathione and other sulfhydryl-containing compounds and then enzymatically converted into 6-thiouric acid, 6-methyl-mercaptopurine, and 6-thioguanine [38]. Ultimately, azathioprine is incorporated into replicating DNA and can block the de novo pathway of purine synthesis. It is this action that is thought to contribute to its relative specificity to lymphocytes due to lack of a salvage pathway. The inhibition of purine synthesis, leads to less DNA and RNA available for the synthesis of white blood cells, including cells of the immune system. Actively replicating cells, such as T cells and B cells of the immune system, which actively synthesize purine to make new DNA are strongly affected [39, 40]. Thus, immunosuppression ensues. It has been used successfully in SLE as steroid sparing agent and in cases of lupus flares. It can be used safely during pregnancy [41]. It can be used as maintenance treatment in lupus nephritis [42].

2.3.2 Methotrexate

If the disease is not controlled with up to 5 mg prednisone methotrexate can be used as an immunosuppressant and steroid sparing agent [43, 44]. Methotrexate exerts anti-inflammatory actions through some well-known and other less well-known mechanisms [45, 46]. It inhibits dihydrofolate reductase thus diminishing the de novo synthesis of purines and pyrimidines by preventing the regeneration from dihydrofolate of tetrahydrofolate. Tetrahydrofolate is essential for the generation of folate cofactors required for purine and pyrimidine synthesis [47]. The reduction in the levels of methyl donors, such as tetrahydrofolate and methyl tetrahydrofolate, by the inhibition of dihydrofolate reductase results in the inhibition of the generation of lymphotoxin polyamines through methionine and S-adenosylmethionine. The inhibition of amino-imidazole-carboxamido-ribonucleotide transformylase results in an increase in intracellular amino-imidazole-carboxamido-ribonucleotide levels. This increase has potent inhibitory effects on AMP deaminase and adenosine deaminase. Thus, adenosine is accumulated. Adenosine confers anti-inflammatory effects [48, 49]. Methotrexate has favorable effects on the joints and the skin [50]. It is teratogenic, therefore if pregnancy is contemplated it should be withdrawn before conception [51].

2.3.3 Mycophenolate mofetil

Mycophenolate mofetil (MMF) has been used for many years in the treatment of SLE. It is a potent immunosuppressing agent with efficacy in lupus nephritis [52] (**Figure 2**) and non-renal lupus [53]. It is particularly indicated in patients with lupus nephritis [54]. MMF is an inhibitor of purine synthesis and it acts to inhibit lymphocyte proliferation and nitric oxide production by activated macrophages [55]. MMF is a prodrug of mycophenolic acid. Mycophenolic acid is an inhibitor of inosine-5'-mononophosphate dehydrogenase [55], it depletes guanosine nucleotides preferentially in T and B lymphocytes and inhibits their proliferation, thereby suppressing cell-mediated immune responses and antibody formation, it inhibits the glycosylation and expression of adhesion molecules, and the recruitment of lymphocytes and monocytes into sites of inflammation, it depletes tetrahydrobiopterin and decreases the production of nitric oxide by inducible NO synthase without affecting the activity of constitutive NO synthases. By these mechanisms MMF exerts anti-inflammatory activity [55]. MMF quickly and persistently reduces numbers of activated B cells and levels of free immunoglobulin light chains [56]. Careful studies in lupus nephritis have established the equivalence of MMF to intravenous (I.V.) cyclophosphamide and its equivalence or superiority to azathioprine in the maintenance phase of treatment [Aspreva Lupus Management Study (ALMS), (MAINTAIN) trial] [57–61]. MMF is effective in non-renal lupus as well. In a systematic review of 20 case series and open-label trials MMF was shown to benefit patients with hematological manifestations and refractory dermatological involvement [62]. It has also been shown to improve lupus arthritis. MMF has side effects including gastrointestinal symptoms, bone marrow suppression, infection risk and long-term risk of cancer from immunosuppression. It appears to be less toxic than cyclophosphamide. Cases of drug sensitivity to MMF have been reported among an Asian subgroup of patients when combined with high-dose corticosteroids [62–64]. By contrast, MMF appears to be more effective in preventing renal flares in high-risk populations such as African Americans [65].

2.3.4 Cyclophosphamide

Cyclophosphamide is an alkylating agent. It crosslinks DNA and results in the death of activated lymphocytes and protects glomeruli [56, 66]. It modulates the expression of T and B cell activation markers [67]. It has been demonstrated in a meta-analysis that there is a decreased risk of end-stage renal disease when cyclophosphamide is applied as standard of care therapy for lupus nephritis [68]. Cyclophosphamide has potential side effects, which include leukopenia, infection risk, bladder toxicity and increased risk of malignancy [69]. Consequently, cyclophosphamide is used as an induction treatment for severe lupus [64, 70] and is replaced by other agents, such as MMF and azathioprine for long-term maintenance treatment.

2.3.5 Calcineurin inhibitors

The use of calcineurin inhibitors tacrolimus and cyclosporin A in SLE is derived from the experience of these drugs gained in organ transplantation. These drugs suppress the production of cytokines, inhibit T- and B cell activation and preserve the renal podocyte actin cytoskeleton, thus reducing proteinuria [71]. In non-renal SLE cyclosporin A exhibits steroid-sparing effects, reduces disease activity and flares [72]. Cyclosporin A acts by modulating lymphocyte function [73, 74]. It forms a complex with cyclophilin to block the phosphatase activity of calcineurin. Thus, it decreases the production of inflammatory cytokines by T lymphocytes [75]. Tacrolimus is preferentially used for lupus nephritis as it exhibits fewer side effects and is characterized by better long-term outcome [76]. Tacrolimus is a macrolide antibiotic with immunosuppressive properties. It has a mode of action similar to that of cyclosporin A, although the two drugs are structurally unrelated. It exerts its effects principally through impairment of gene expression in target cells [77]. Tacrolimus bonds to an immunophilin and this complex inhibits calcineurin phosphatase. Tacrolimus inhibits calcium-dependent events, such as interleukin-2 gene transcription, nitric oxide synthase activation, cell degranulation, and apoptosis. It also potentiates the actions of glucocorticoids. It may enhance expression of the transforming growth factor beta-1 gene [78]. T cell proliferation, especially type 1 T helper cell, in response to ligation of the T cell receptor is inhibited by tacrolimus. Tacrolimus has been successfully applied in combination with low-dose MMF and corticosteroids as induction therapy in lupus nephritis [76, 79, 80]. Tacrolimus (0.075 mg/kg/day) has been used in refractory lupus nephritis with good results [81], however severe drug adverse events were observed, such as a high rate of infections and diabetic ketoacidosis. Cyclosporin A (2.6-3.7 mg/kg/day) has also been used in refractory lupus nephritis with good results, however drug adverse events such as tremor and hypertension have been noted [81]. Voclosporin, a novel calcineurin inhibitor is now used in lupus nephritis and is showing promising results [82].

2.3.6 Plasmapheresis

Plasmapheresis has been used successfully in refractory cases of neuropsychiatric lupus [83]. Plasmapheresis has also been applied in pregnant women with active lupus or antiphospholipid syndrome or in cases of lupus nephritis [84]. Immunoadsorption, is replacing plasmapheresis and appears to have good results [84].

2.3.7 Intravenous immunoglobulin

Therapeutic intravenous immunoglobulin (IV IG) mostly consists of human polyspecific immunoglobulin G. IV IG has been used in patients with systemic lupus erythematosus and was shown to reduce the activity of the disease [85]. IV IG may be used in cases of refractory neuropsychiatric lupus [83] and in lupus myocarditis [86].

2.4 Biologics

Biologic drugs currently incorporated in SLE treatment are rituximab [87–89] and belimumab [90–93] (**Figure 1**). The sequential use of rituximab and belimumab is also under investigation [94, 95]. Other biologic agents targeting the B lymphocyte have also been applied [96]. Various biologic drugs have been used in treatment regimens for SLE patients with poor response or side effects to standard treatment [97]. The original goal of biologics was to induce disease remission and establish self-tolerance [98, 99]. This goal has not been achieved. It may be that the heterogeneity of disease mechanisms inherent in SLE may guide the introduction of cell- and cytokine- or pathway specific therapies which will be effective in various subgroups of SLE patients [97].

2.4.1 Rituximab

Rituximab is a humanized anti-CD20 monoclonal antibody used for B cell depletion therapy. Rituximab can induce killing of CD20+ cells via various mechanisms.

The effects of rituximab include complement-mediated cytotoxicity and antibody-dependent cell-mediated cytotoxicity [100]. Targeting the B cell has been proposed by many research studies in SLE [101]. Results from various registries have shown a favorable benefit-risk ratio in treatment refractory SLE [102, 103]. Rituximab has been shown to be safe and effective in the treatment of non-renal SLE [103]. Namely, it decreases disease activity, immunologic parameters and has a steroid-sparing effect. It can be recommended for organ-specific manifestations, such as arthritis and thrombocytopenia. Rituximab has been shown to be effective for certain refractory SLE patients, in particular refractory neuropsychiatric SLE [104]. Thus, it can be administered in this patient group. The therapeutic effect of rituximab has been compared with that of MMF and with that of cyclophosphamide in a trial of 54 lupus nephritis patients and was shown to be equally effective [105]. B cell depletion is observed but it is not complete, because early B cells and plasma cells do not express CD20 [106]. Normalization of B cell subsets has been observed in rituximab-treated SLE patients [101]. In the initial introduction of rituximab, it was suggested that complete B cell depletion might confer a better outcome for SLE [101]. However, SLE flares were observed after repeated rituximab infusions. These flares were thought to be a result of elevated circulating CD257 (BLyS) levels and high anti-dsDNA levels [107, 108]. Thus, it was proposed that B cell depletion with rituximab induced a surge in CD257 levels that may have exacerbated disease in some SLE patients [106]. In these individuals, rituximab depletion was followed by rapid peripheral B cell reconstitution, with increased circulating plasmablasts. It has been suggested that these plasmablasts might stimulate autoreactive T helper cells, which promote autoantibody production and may drive a positive feedback loop promoting disease activity [106]. Consequently, rituximab is considered in lupus nephritis only after cyclophosphamide and MMF have failed or in relapses [109]. Despite that, an analysis of the LUNAR study showed complete response with rituximab in cases of lupus nephritis [110].

2.4.2 Belimumab

Belimumab, the anti-CD257 monoclonal antibody, acts as a soluble CD257 antagonist and was the first drug approved in more than 50 years by the FDA for SLE [111–118]. The recognition of B cells as central in the pathogenesis of SLE led to the development of drugs that block B cells, including antibodies to B-cell surface antigens, B-cell tolerogens, blockers of co-stimulatory molecules and inhibitors of cytokines with direct effect on B cells [119]. The BAFF/APRIL axis has been thoroughly investigated as these cytokines are vital to B-cell maturation and survival [115, 120, 121]. Belimumab is an anti-BAFF antibody. Belimumab should be considered in extrarenal lupus in patients with inadequate response to hydrochloroquine and corticosteroids and immunosuppressive drugs [122]. Patients with cutaneous and musculoskeletal manifestations are expected to respond better. Belimumab was tested in a study in which it was administered in lupus patients after rituximab [123]. The effects of belimumab on proteinuria and neuropsychiatric SLE were examined in a recent study. It was found that belimumab decreased proteinuria and improved neuropsychiatric symptoms in neuropsychiatric SLE [124]. The US Food and Drug Administration (FDA) has expanded the indication for belimumab to adults with active lupus nephritis who are receiving standard therapy. The expanded indication for belimumab for patients with LN is based on findings from the BLISS-LN phase 3 trial. In this randomized placebo controlled clinical trial on the effect of belimumab on lupus nephritis it was shown that belimumab led more patients to a primary efficacy renal response than placebo and also led to a complete renal response more patients than the placebo [125]. The risk of a renal related event or death was lower among patients receiving belimumab.

2.4.3 Obinutuzumab

Obinutuzumab is a novel humanized type II glycoengineered anti-CD20 antibody [126]. In vitro studies have shown that obinutuzumab may induce superior B cell cytotoxicity as compared to rituximab in patients with SLE [126]. Obinutuzumab is considered an alternative B-cell depleting agent for the treatment of SLE [127]. It has been suggested that SLE patients with secondary non-response to rituximab should be preferentially switched to another B-cell depleting agent instead of belimumab [128].

2.4.4 Ofatumumab

Ofatumumab is a fully human anti-CD20 monoclonal antibody [129]. It induces antibody-dependent cell-mediated cytotoxicity and complement-dependent cytotoxicity in CD20-expressing B lymphocytes. Ofatumumab is highly potent in lysing B cells, as this appears to stem from its binding site on the short extracellular loop of the target CD20 protein and its slow release from the target molecule. Ofatumumab has been successfully applied in a patient with SLE and hypocomplementemia in combination with fresh frozen plasma [130]. Ofatumumab, has been used as B cell depleting therapy in SLE patients who developed severe infusion reactions to rituximab [131]. The agent was well tolerated and may be a safe and effective alternative to rituximab for B cell depletion treatment in SLE.

2.4.5 Epratuzumab

Epratuzumab is a humanized monoclonal antibody [132]. It targets CD22 on B cells and acts as B-cell modulating treatment through inhibition of B-cell receptor signaling. It has been applied in SLE [133] and found to be effective in SLE patients with Sjogren's syndrome [134].

2.4.6 Sifalimumab

Interferons (IFNs) are a family of potent immunostimulatory cytokines that are broadly divided into three subtypes, type I, type II and type III [135]. Of all the type I IFNs, IFNα is the most abundant and is well characterized. The role of interferons in autoimmunity, especially SLE is discussed [136]. Sifalimumab is a fully human monoclonal antibody against multiple IFN-α subtypes and has shown promise in a phase IIb clinical trial in SLE [137].

2.4.7 Rigerimod

Rigerimod is a peptide which reduces the stability of MHC molecules that present antigens to T cells, thus blocking antigen presentation to autoreactive T cells thereby blocking B cell maturation. It has been tested in SLE patients with encouraging results [138].

2.5 Supplementary therapeutic modalities

Recently efforts have been made to incorporate adjunct therapeutic agents in the treatment of SLE, so, as to reduce the toxicity of traditional drugs. Prasterone and vitamin D are two immunomodulatory agents, which have been applied in the treatment of SLE as supplements, in order to control disease activity and reduce the use of corticosteroids. Prasterone is a synthetic form of the hormone dehydroepiandrosterone [139]. Its use led SLE patients to better tolerate the tapering of corticosteroids [140] and stabilized disease activity in some patients [141]. Vitamin D has immunomodulatory properties, namely it decreases inflammatory cytokines and down regulates the renin-angiotensin system [142, 143]. It may lead to the improvement of disease activity in SLE, as shown by some but not all studies [144–146].

3. Therapeutic strategies for the management of SLE

In 2014 a panel of experts introduced the treating-to-target approach in the management of SLE [147]. In 2019 an update of the EULAR recommendations for the management of SLE was published [148]. These recommendations are based both on evidence as well as on expert opinion. According to these recommendations, hydroxychloroquine should be administered to all lupus patients at a dose not exceeding 5 mg/kg real body weight. During chronic maintenance therapy glucocorticoids should be minimized to less than 7.5 mg/day and withdrawn if possible. Initiation of immunomodulatory agents can aid in tapering or withdrawal of corticosteroids. In active or flaring extra-renal disease belimumab should be considered. Rituximab is an option for organ-threatening refractory disease. Various approaches for the treatment of SLE are currently under investigation. These include various methods to target interferon I, such as the use of anifrolumab, a human monoclonal antidoy to type I interferon receptor subunit 1 [149, 150], and to inhibit T cell co-stimulation [151]. Baricitinib, an oral selective Janus kinase1 and Janus kinase 2 inhibitor is an oral treatment, which was tested in SLE patients with favorable results [152].

4. Conclusion

Hydroxychloroquine and prednisone remain standard of care treatment for SLE. When flares occur the introduction of immunosuppressive agents and/or biologic drugs improves disease activity and disease outcome in SLE. Nowadays, the introduction of biologic agents, such as rituximab and belimumab have revolutionized the treatment of SLE and have opened new therapeutic horizons in all the spectrum of lupus disease.

Author details

Panagiotis Athanassiou[1*], Lambros Athanassiou[2] and
Ifigenia Kostoglou-Athanassiou[3]

1 Department of Rheumatology, St. Paul's Hospital, Thessaloniki, Greece

2 Department of Rheumatology, Asclepeion Hospital, Voula, Athens, Greece

3 Department of Endocrinology, Asclepeion Hospital, Voula, Athens, Greece

*Address all correspondence to: pathanassiou@yahoo.gr

References

[1] Ben-Zvi I, Kivity S, Langevitz P, Shoenfeld Y. Hydroxychloroquine: from malaria to autoimmunity. *Clin Rev Allergy Immunol*. Apr 2012;42(2):145-53. doi:10.1007/s12016-010-8243-x

[2] Hu C, Lu L, Wan JP, Wen C. The Pharmacological Mechanisms and Therapeutic Activities of Hydroxychloroquine in Rheumatic and Related Diseases. *Curr Med Chem*. 2017;24(20): 2241-2249. doi:10.2174/0929867324666170316115938

[3] Rynes RI. Antimalarial drugs in the treatment of rheumatological diseases. *Br J Rheumatol*. Jul 1997;36(7):799-805. doi:10.1093/rheumatology/36.7.799

[4] Rainsford KD, Parke AL, Clifford-Rashotte M, Kean WF. Therapy and pharmacological properties of hydroxychloroquine and chloroquine in treatment of systemic lupus erythematosus, rheumatoid arthritis and related diseases. *Inflammopharmacology*. Oct 2015;23(5):231-69. doi:10.1007/s10787-015-0239-y

[5] James JA, Kim-Howard XR, Bruner BF, et al. Hydroxychloroquine sulfate treatment is associated with later onset of systemic lupus erythematosus. *Lupus*. 2007;16(6):401-9. doi:10.1177/s0961203307078579

[6] Fischer-Betz R, Schneider M. [Antimalarials. A treatment option for every lupus patient!?]. *Z Rheumatol*. Sep 2009;68(7):584, 586-90. Antimalariamittel: Therapieoption für jeden Lupus-Patienten?! doi:10.1007/s00393-008-0412-4

[7] Fox RI. Mechanism of action of hydroxychloroquine as an antirheumatic drug. *Semin Arthritis Rheum*. Oct 1993;23(2 Suppl 1):82-91. doi:10.1016/s0049-0172(10)80012-5

[8] Fox R. Anti-malarial drugs: possible mechanisms of action in autoimmune disease and prospects for drug development. *Lupus*. Jun 1996;5 Suppl 1:S4-10.

[9] Schrezenmeier E, Dörner T. Mechanisms of action of hydroxychloroquine and chloroquine: implications for rheumatology. *Nat Rev Rheumatol*. Mar 2020;16(3):155-166. doi:10.1038/s41584-020-0372-x

[10] Ruiz-Irastorza G, Ramos-Casals M, Brito-Zeron P, Khamashta MA. Clinical efficacy and side effects of antimalarials in systemic lupus erythematosus: a systematic review. *Ann Rheum Dis*. Jan 2010;69(1):20-8. doi:10.1136/ard.2008.101766

[11] Floris A, Piga M, Mangoni AA, Bortoluzzi A, Erre GL, Cauli A. Protective Effects of Hydroxychloroquine against Accelerated Atherosclerosis in Systemic Lupus Erythematosus. *Mediators Inflamm*. 2018;2018:3424136. doi:10.1155/2018/3424136

[12] Penn SK, Kao AH, Schott LL, et al. Hydroxychloroquine and glycemia in women with rheumatoid arthritis and systemic lupus erythematosus. *J Rheumatol*. Jun 2010;37(6):1136-42. doi:10.3899/jrheum.090994

[13] Ruiz-Irastorza G, Khamashta MA. Hydroxychloroquine: the cornerstone of lupus therapy. *Lupus*. 2008:271-3. vol. 4.

[14] Babary H, Liu X, Ayatollahi Y, et al. Favorable effects of hydroxychloroquine on serum low density lipid in patients with systemic lupus erythematosus: A systematic review and meta-analysis. *Int J Rheum Dis*. Jan 2018;21(1):84-92. doi:10.1111/1756-185x.13159

[15] Qiao X, Zhou ZC, Niu R, et al. Hydroxychloroquine Improves Obesity-Associated Insulin Resistance and Hepatic Steatosis by Regulating Lipid Metabolism. *Front Pharmacol*. 2019;10:855. doi:10.3389/fphar.2019.00855

[16] Morris SJ, Wasko MC, Antohe JL, et al. Hydroxychloroquine use associated with improvement in lipid profiles in rheumatoid arthritis patients. *Arthritis Care Res (Hoboken)*. Apr 2011;63(4): 530-4. doi:10.1002/acr.20393

[17] Petri M. Use of hydroxychloroquine to prevent thrombosis in systemic lupus erythematosus and in antiphospholipid antibody-positive patients. *Curr Rheumatol Rep*. Feb 2011;13(1):77-80. doi:10.1007/s11926-010-0141-y

[18] Pareek A, Chandurkar N, Thomas N, et al. Efficacy and safety of hydroxychloroquine in the treatment of type 2 diabetes mellitus: a double blind, randomized comparison with pioglitazone. *Curr Med Res Opin*. Jul 2014; 30(7):1257-66. doi:10.1185/03007995.2014.909393

[19] Kasturi S, Sammaritano LR. Corticosteroids in Lupus. *Rheum Dis Clin North Am*. Feb 2016;42(1):47-62, viii. doi:10.1016/j.rdc.2015.08.007

[20] Ugarte A, Danza A, Ruiz-Irastorza G. Glucocorticoids and antimalarials in systemic lupus erythematosus: an update and future directions. *Curr Opin Rheumatol*. Sep 2018;30(5):482-489. doi:10.1097/bor.0000000000000527

[21] Vandewalle J, Luypaert A, De Bosscher K, Libert C. Therapeutic Mechanisms of Glucocorticoids. *Trends Endocrinol Metab*. Jan 2018;29(1):42-54. doi:10.1016/j.tem.2017.10.010

[22] Dasgupta S. Therapeutic Interventions of Tissue Specific Autoimmune Onset in Systemic Lupus Erythematosus. *Mini Rev Med Chem*. 2017;17(15):1418-1424. doi:10.2174/1389557516666160611020838

[23] Strehl C, Ehlers L, Gaber T, Buttgereit F. Glucocorticoids-All-Rounders Tackling the Versatile Players of the Immune System. *Front Immunol*. 2019;10:1744. doi:10.3389/fimmu.2019.01744

[24] Newton R, Holden NS. Separating transrepression and transactivation: a distressing divorce for the glucocorticoid receptor? *Mol Pharmacol*. Oct 2007;72(4):799-809. doi:10.1124/mol.107.038794

[25] Danza A, Ruiz-Irastorza G. Infection risk in systemic lupus erythematosus patients: susceptibility factors and preventive strategies. *Lupus*. Oct 2013;22(12):1286-94. doi:10.1177/0961203313493032

[26] Yates DJ, Mon SY, Oh Y, et al. Multicentre retrospective cohort study assessing the incidence of serious infections in patients with lupus nephritis, compared with non-renal systemic lupus erythematosus. *Lupus Sci Med*. Sep 2020;7(1)doi:10.1136/lupus-2020-000390

[27] Ruiz-Arruza I, Ugarte A, Cabezas-Rodriguez I, Medina JA, Moran MA, Ruiz-Irastorza G. Glucocorticoids and irreversible damage in patients with systemic lupus erythematosus. *Rheumatology (Oxford)*. Aug 2014;53(8):1470-6. doi:10.1093/rheumatology/keu148

[28] Zonana-Nacach A, Barr SG, Magder LS, Petri M. Damage in systemic lupus erythematosus and its association with corticosteroids. *Arthritis Rheum*. Aug 2000;43(8):1801-8. doi:10.1002/1529-0131(200008)43:8<1801::aid-anr16>3.0.co;2-o

[29] Ruiz-Irastorza G, Ugarte A, Saint-Pastou Terrier C, et al. Repeated pulses of methyl-prednisolone with reduced doses of prednisone improve the outcome of class III, IV and V lupus nephritis: An observational comparative study of the Lupus-Cruces and lupus-Bordeaux cohorts. *Autoimmun Rev*. Aug 2017;16(8):826-832. doi:10.1016/j.autrev.2017.05.017

[30] Mosca M, Neri R, Giannessi S, et al. Therapy with pulse methylprednisolone

and short course pulse cyclophosphamide for diffuse proliferative glomerulonephritis. *Lupus*. 2001;10(4):253-7. doi:10.1191/096120301680416931

[31] Badsha H, Edwards CJ. Intravenous pulses of methylprednisolone for systemic lupus erythematosus. *Semin Arthritis Rheum*. Jun 2003;32(6):370-7. doi:10.1053/sarh.2002.50003

[32] Badsha H, Kong KO, Lian TY, Chan SP, Edwards CJ, Chng HH. Low-dose pulse methylprednisolone for systemic lupus erythematosus flares is efficacious and has a decreased risk of infectious complications. *Lupus*. 2002;11(8):508-13. doi:10.1191/0961203302lu243oa

[33] Roccatello D, Sciascia S, Rossi D, et al. Intensive short-term treatment with rituximab, cyclophosphamide and methylprednisolone pulses induces remission in severe cases of SLE with nephritis and avoids further immunosuppressive maintenance therapy. *Nephrol Dial Transplant*. Dec 2011;26(12):3987-92. doi:10.1093/ndt/gfr109

[34] Ruiz-Arruza I, Barbosa C, Ugarte A, Ruiz-Irastorza G. Comparison of high versus low-medium prednisone doses for the treatment of systemic lupus erythematosus patients with high activity at diagnosis. *Autoimmun Rev*. Oct 2015;14(10):875-9. doi:10.1016/j.autrev.2015.05.011

[35] Mathian A, Pha M, Haroche J, et al. Withdrawal of low-dose prednisone in SLE patients with a clinically quiescent disease for more than 1 year: a randomised clinical trial. *Ann Rheum Dis*. Mar 2020;79(3):339-346. doi:10.1136/annrheumdis-2019-216303

[36] van Vollenhoven R, Voskuyl A, Bertsias G, et al. A framework for remission in SLE: consensus findings from a large international task force on definitions of remission in SLE (DORIS). *Ann Rheum Dis*. Mar 2017;76(3):554-561. doi:10.1136/annrheumdis-2016-209519

[37] Abu-Shakra M, Shoenfeld Y. Azathioprine therapy for patients with systemic lupus erythematosus. *Lupus*. 2001;10(3):152-3. doi:10.1191/096120301676669495

[38] Aarbakke J, Janka-Schaub G, Elion GB. Thiopurine biology and pharmacology. *Trends Pharmacol Sci*. 1997:3-7. vol. 1.

[39] Patel AA, Swerlick RA, McCall CO. Azathioprine in dermatology: the past, the present, and the future. *J Am Acad Dermatol*. Sep 2006;55(3):369-89. doi:10.1016/j.jaad.2005.07.059

[40] Maltzman JS, Koretzky GA. Azathioprine: old drug, new actions. *J Clin Invest*. Apr 2003;111(8):1122-4. doi:10.1172/jci18384

[41] Saavedra M, Sánchez A, Morales S, Ángeles U, Jara LJ. Azathioprine during pregnancy in systemic lupus erythematosus patients is not associated with poor fetal outcome. *Clin Rheumatol*. Jul 2015;34(7):1211-6. doi:10.1007/s10067-015-2987-x

[42] Jaryal A, Vikrant S. Current status of lupus nephritis. *Indian J Med Res*. Feb 2017;145(2):167-178. doi:10.4103/ijmr.IJMR_163_16

[43] Fortin PR, Abrahamowicz M, Ferland D, Lacaille D, Smith CD, Zummer M. Steroid-sparing effects of methotrexate in systemic lupus erythematosus: a double-blind, randomized, placebo-controlled trial. *Arthritis Rheum*. Dec 15 2008;59(12):1796-804. doi:10.1002/art.24068

[44] Muangchan C, van Vollenhoven RF, Bernatsky SR, et al. Treatment Algorithms in Systemic Lupus Erythematosus. *Arthritis Care Res (Hoboken)*. Sep 2015;67(9):1237-1245. doi:10.1002/acr.22589

[45] Chan ES, Cronstein BN. Mechanisms of action of methotrexate. *Bull Hosp Jt Dis (2013)*. 2013;71 Suppl 1:S5-8.

[46] Cronstein BN, Aune TM. Methotrexate and its mechanisms of action in inflammatory arthritis. *Nat Rev Rheumatol*. Mar 2020;16(3):145-154. doi:10.1038/s41584-020-0373-9

[47] Bedoui Y, Guillot X, Sélambarom J, et al. Methotrexate an Old Drug with New Tricks. *Int J Mol Sci*. Oct 10 2019;20(20)doi:10.3390/ijms20205023

[48] Cronstein BN. The mechanism of action of methotrexate. *Rheum Dis Clin North Am*. Nov 1997;23(4):739-55. doi:10.1016/s0889-857x(05)70358-6

[49] Chan ES, Cronstein BN. Methotrexate--how does it really work? *Nat Rev Rheumatol*. 2010:175-8.

[50] Bertsias G, Ioannidis JP, Boletis J, et al. EULAR recommendations for the management of systemic lupus erythematosus. Report of a Task Force of the EULAR Standing Committee for International Clinical Studies Including Therapeutics. *Ann Rheum Dis*. Feb 2008;67(2):195-205. doi:10.1136/ard.2007.070367

[51] Vroom F, de Walle HE, van de Laar MA, Brouwers JR, de Jong-van den Berg LT. Disease-modifying antirheumatic drugs in pregnancy: current status and implications for the future. *Drug Saf*. 2006;29(10):845-63. doi:10.2165/00002018-200629100-00003

[52] Walsh M, James M, Jayne D, Tonelli M, Manns BJ, Hemmelgarn BR. Mycophenolate mofetil for induction therapy of lupus nephritis: a systematic review and meta-analysis. *Clin J Am Soc Nephrol*. Sep 2007;2(5):968-75. doi:10.2215/cjn.01200307

[53] Pisoni CN, Karim Y, Cuadrado MJ. Mycophenolate mofetil and systemic lupus erythematosus: an overview. *Lupus*. 2005;14 Suppl 1:s9-11. doi:10.1191/0961203305lu2111oa

[54] Joo YB, Kang YM, Kim HA, et al. Outcome and predictors of renal survival in patients with lupus nephritis: Comparison between cyclophosphamide and mycophenolate mofetil. *Int J Rheum Dis*. May 2018;21(5):1031-1039. doi:10.1111/1756-185x.13274

[55] Allison AC. Mechanisms of action of mycophenolate mofetil. *Lupus*. 2005;14 Suppl 1:s2-8. doi:10.1191/0961203305lu2109oa

[56] Fassbinder T, Saunders U, Mickholz E, et al. Differential effects of cyclophosphamide and mycophenolate mofetil on cellular and serological parameters in patients with systemic lupus erythematosus. *Arthritis Res Ther*. Apr 3 2015;17(1):92. doi:10.1186/s13075-015-0603-8

[57] Morris HK, Canetta PA, Appel GB. Impact of the ALMS and MAINTAIN trials on the management of lupus nephritis. *Nephrol Dial Transplant*. Jun 2013;28(6):1371-6. doi:10.1093/ndt/gfs447

[58] Sinclair A, Appel G, Dooley MA, et al. Mycophenolate mofetil as induction and maintenance therapy for lupus nephritis: rationale and protocol for the randomized, controlled Aspreva Lupus Management Study (ALMS). *Lupus*. 2007;16(12):972-80. doi:10.1177/0961203307084712

[59] Houssiau FA, D'Cruz D, Sangle S, et al. Azathioprine versus mycophenolate mofetil for long-term immunosuppression in lupus nephritis: results from the MAINTAIN Nephritis Trial. *Ann Rheum Dis*. Dec 2010;69(12):2083-9. doi:10.1136/ard.2010.131995

[60] Stoenoiu MS, Aydin S, Tektonidou M, et al. Repeat kidney biopsies fail to detect differences between azathioprine and mycophenolate mofetil

maintenance therapy for lupus nephritis: data from the MAINTAIN Nephritis Trial. *Nephrol Dial Transplant*. May 2012;27(5):1924-30. doi:10.1093/ndt/gfr553

[61] Ginzler EM, Wofsy D, Isenberg D, Gordon C, Lisk L, Dooley MA. Nonrenal disease activity following mycophenolate mofetil or intravenous cyclophosphamide as induction treatment for lupus nephritis: findings in a multicenter, prospective, randomized, open-label, parallel-group clinical trial. *Arthritis Rheum*. Jan 2010;62(1):211-21. doi:10.1002/art.25052

[62] Mok CC. Mycophenolate mofetil for non-renal manifestations of systemic lupus erythematosus: a systematic review. *Scand J Rheumatol*. Sep-Oct 2007;36(5):329-37. doi:10.1080/03009740701607042

[63] Appel GB, Contreras G, Dooley MA, et al. Mycophenolate mofetil versus cyclophosphamide for induction treatment of lupus nephritis. *J Am Soc Nephrol*. May 2009;20(5):1103-12. doi:10.1681/asn.2008101028

[64] Houssiau FA, Vasconcelos C, D'Cruz D, et al. The 10-year follow-up data of the Euro-Lupus Nephritis Trial comparing low-dose and high-dose intravenous cyclophosphamide. *Ann Rheum Dis*. Jan 2010;69(1):61-4. doi:10.1136/ard.2008.102533

[65] Yap DY, Chan TM. Lupus Nephritis in Asia: Clinical Features and Management. *Kidney Dis (Basel)*. Sep 2015;1(2):100-9. doi:10.1159/000430458

[66] Hurd ER, Ziff M. The mechanism of action of cyclophosphamide on the nephritis of (NZB x NZW)F1 hybrid mice. *Clin Exp Immunol*. Jul 1977;29(1):132-9.

[67] Amano H, Morimoto S, Kaneko H, Tokano Y, Takasaki Y, Hashimoto H. Effect of intravenous cyclophosphamide in systemic lupus erythematosus: relation to lymphocyte subsets and activation markers. *Lupus*. 2000;9(1):26-32. doi:10.1177/096120330000900106

[68] Koo HS, Kim YC, Lee SW, et al. The effects of cyclophosphamide and mycophenolate on end-stage renal disease and death of lupus nephritis. *Lupus*. Nov 2011;20(13):1442-9. doi:10.1177/0961203311416034

[69] Martin F, Lauwerys B, Lefèbvre C, Devogelaer JP, Houssiau FA. Side-effects of intravenous cyclophosphamide pulse therapy. *Lupus*. 1997;6(3):254-7. doi:10.1177/096120339700600307

[70] Houssiau FA, Vasconcelos C, D'Cruz D, et al. Immunosuppressive therapy in lupus nephritis: the Euro-Lupus Nephritis Trial, a randomized trial of low-dose versus high-dose intravenous cyclophosphamide. *Arthritis Rheum*. Aug 2002;46(8):2121-31. doi:10.1002/art.10461

[71] Faul C, Donnelly M, Merscher-Gomez S, et al. The actin cytoskeleton of kidney podocytes is a direct target of the antiproteinuric effect of cyclosporine A. *Nat Med*. Sep 2008;14(9):931-8. doi:10.1038/nm.1857

[72] Pego-Reigosa JM, Cobo-Ibáñez T, Calvo-Alén J, et al. Efficacy and safety of nonbiologic immunosuppressants in the treatment of nonrenal systemic lupus erythematosus: a systematic review. *Arthritis Care Res (Hoboken)*. Nov 2013;65(11):1775-85. doi:10.1002/acr.22035

[73] Schreiber SL, Crabtree GR. The mechanism of action of cyclosporin A and FK506. *Immunol Today*. Apr 1992;13(4):136-42. doi:10.1016/0167-5699(92)90111-j

[74] Russell G, Graveley R, Seid J, al-Humidan AK, Skjodt H. Mechanisms of action of cyclosporine and effects on

connective tissues. *Semin Arthritis Rheum*. Jun 1992;21(6 Suppl 3):16-22. doi:10.1016/0049-0172(92)90009-3

[75] Matsuda S, Koyasu S. Mechanisms of action of cyclosporine. *Immunopharmacology*. May 2000;47(2-3):119-25. doi:10.1016/s0162-3109(00)00192-2

[76] Mok CC. Towards new avenues in the management of lupus glomerulonephritis. *Nat Rev Rheumatol*. Apr 2016;12(4):221-34. doi:10.1038/nrrheum.2015.174

[77] Thomson AW, Bonham CA, Zeevi A. Mode of action of tacrolimus (FK506): molecular and cellular mechanisms. *Ther Drug Monit*. Dec 1995;17(6):584-91. doi:10.1097/00007691-199512000-00007

[78] Yoon KH. Efficacy and cytokine modulating effects of tacrolimus in systemic lupus erythematosus: a review. *J Biomed Biotechnol*. 2010;2010:686480. doi:10.1155/2010/686480

[79] Bao H, Liu ZH, Xie HL, Hu WX, Zhang HT, Li LS. Successful treatment of class V+IV lupus nephritis with multitarget therapy. *J Am Soc Nephrol*. Oct 2008;19(10):2001-10. doi:10.1681/asn.2007121272

[80] Liu Z, Zhang H, Xing C, et al. Multitarget therapy for induction treatment of lupus nephritis: a randomized trial. *Ann Intern Med*. Jan 6 2015;162(1):18-26. doi:10.7326/m14-1030

[81] Kronbichler A, Brezina B, Gauckler P, Quintana LF, Jayne DRW. Refractory lupus nephritis: When, why and how to treat. *Autoimmun Rev*. May 2019;18(5):510-518. doi:10.1016/j.autrev.2019.03.004

[82] Rovin BH, Solomons N, Pendergraft WF, 3rd, et al. A randomized, controlled double-blind study comparing the efficacy and safety of dose-ranging voclosporin with placebo in achieving remission in patients with active lupus nephritis. *Kidney Int*. Jan 2019;95(1):219-231. doi:10.1016/j.kint.2018.08.025

[83] Magro-Checa C, Zirkzee EJ, Huizinga TW, Steup-Beekman GM. Management of Neuropsychiatric Systemic Lupus Erythematosus: Current Approaches and Future Perspectives. *Drugs*. Mar 2016;76(4):459-83. doi:10.1007/s40265-015-0534-3

[84] Kronbichler A, Brezina B, Quintana LF, Jayne DR. Efficacy of plasma exchange and immunoadsorption in systemic lupus erythematosus and antiphospholipid syndrome: A systematic review. *Autoimmun Rev*. Jan 2016;15(1):38-49. doi:10.1016/j.autrev.2015.08.010

[85] Sakthiswary R, D'Cruz D. Intravenous immunoglobulin in the therapeutic armamentarium of systemic lupus erythematosus: a systematic review and meta-analysis. *Medicine (Baltimore)*. Oct 2014;93(16):e86. doi:10.1097/md.0000000000000086

[86] Suri V, Varma S, Joshi K, Malhotra P, Kumari S, Jain S. Lupus myocarditis: marked improvement in cardiac function after intravenous immunoglobulin therapy. *Rheumatol Int*. Sep 2010;30(11):1503-5. doi:10.1007/s00296-009-1098-x

[87] Merrill JT, Neuwelt CM, Wallace DJ, et al. Efficacy and safety of rituximab in moderately-to-severely active systemic lupus erythematosus: the randomized, double-blind, phase II/III systemic lupus erythematosus evaluation of rituximab trial. *Arthritis Rheum*. Jan 2010;62(1):222-33. doi:10.1002/art.27233

[88] Pirone C, Mendoza-Pinto C, van der Windt DA, Parker B, M OS, Bruce IN. Predictive and prognostic factors influencing outcomes of rituximab therapy in systemic lupus erythematosus (SLE): A systematic review. *Semin Arthritis Rheum*. Dec

2017;47(3):384-396. doi:10.1016/j.semarthrit.2017.04.010

[89] Iwata S, Saito K, Hirata S, et al. Efficacy and safety of anti-CD20 antibody rituximab for patients with refractory systemic lupus erythematosus. *Lupus*. Apr 2018;27(5):802-811. doi:10.1177/0961203317749047

[90] Navarra SV, Guzmán RM, Gallacher AE, et al. Efficacy and safety of belimumab in patients with active systemic lupus erythematosus: a randomised, placebo-controlled, phase 3 trial. *Lancet*. Feb 26 2011;377(9767):721-31. doi:10.1016/s0140-6736(10)61354-2

[91] Blair HA, Duggan ST. Belimumab: A Review in Systemic Lupus Erythematosus. *Drugs*. Mar 2018;78(3):355-366. doi:10.1007/s40265-018-0872-z

[92] Poh YJ, Baptista B, D'Cruz DP. Subcutaneous and intravenous belimumab in the treatment of systemic lupus erythematosus: a review of data on subcutaneous and intravenous administration. *Expert Rev Clin Immunol*. Oct 2017;13(10):925-938. doi:10.1080/1744666x.2017.1371592

[93] Wallace DJ, Ginzler EM, Merrill JT, et al. Safety and Efficacy of Belimumab Plus Standard Therapy for Up to Thirteen Years in Patients With Systemic Lupus Erythematosus. *Arthritis Rheumatol*. Jul 2019;71(7):1125-1134. doi:10.1002/art.40861

[94] Kraaij T, Kamerling SWA, de Rooij ENM, et al. The NET-effect of combining rituximab with belimumab in severe systemic lupus erythematosus. *J Autoimmun*. Jul 2018;91:45-54. doi:10.1016/j.jaut.2018.03.003

[95] Gualtierotti R, Borghi MO, Gerosa M, et al. Successful sequential therapy with rituximab and belimumab in patients with active systemic lupus erythematosus: a case series. *Clin Exp Rheumatol*. Jul-Aug 2018;36(4):643-647.

[96] Lee WS, Amengual O. B cells targeting therapy in the management of systemic lupus erythematosus. *Immunol Med*. Mar 2020;43(1):16-35. doi:10.1080/25785826.2019.1698929

[97] Davis LS, Reimold AM. Research and therapeutics-traditional and emerging therapies in systemic lupus erythematosus. *Rheumatology (Oxford)*. Apr 1 2017;56(suppl_1):i100-i113. doi:10.1093/rheumatology/kew417

[98] Magro R. Biological therapies and their clinical impact in the treatment of systemic lupus erythematosus. *Ther Adv Musculoskelet Dis*. 2019;11:1759720x19874309. doi:10.1177/1759720x19874309

[99] Samotij D, Reich A. Biologics in the Treatment of Lupus Erythematosus: A Critical Literature Review. *Biomed Res Int*. 2019;2019:8142368. doi:10.1155/2019/8142368

[100] Cerny T, Borisch B, Introna M, Johnson P, Rose AL. Mechanism of action of rituximab. *Anticancer Drugs*. Nov 2002;13 Suppl 2:S3-10. doi:10.1097/00001813-200211002-00002

[101] Sanz I, Lee FE. B cells as therapeutic targets in SLE. *Nat Rev Rheumatol*. Jun 2010;6(6):326-37. doi:10.1038/nrrheum.2010.68

[102] Witt M, Grunke M, Proft F, et al. Clinical outcomes and safety of rituximab treatment for patients with systemic lupus erythematosus (SLE) - results from a nationwide cohort in Germany (GRAID). *Lupus*. Oct 2013;22(11):1142-9. doi:10.1177/0961203313503912

[103] Cobo-Ibáñez T, Loza-Santamaría E, Pego-Reigosa JM, et al. Efficacy and safety of rituximab in the treatment of non-renal systemic lupus erythematosus: a systematic review. *Semin Arthritis Rheum*. Oct 2014;44(2):175-85. doi:10.1016/j.semarthrit.2014.04.002

[104] Tokunaga M, Saito K, Kawabata D, et al. Efficacy of rituximab (anti-CD20) for refractory systemic lupus erythematosus involving the central nervous system. *Ann Rheum Dis*. Apr 2007; 66(4):470-5. doi:10.1136/ard.2006.057885

[105] Moroni G, Raffiotta F, Trezzi B, et al. Rituximab vs mycophenolate and vs cyclophosphamide pulses for induction therapy of active lupus nephritis: a clinical observational study. *Rheumatology (Oxford)*. Sep 2014;53(9):1570-7. doi:10.1093/rheumatology/ket462

[106] Ehrenstein MR, Wing C. The BAFFling effects of rituximab in lupus: danger ahead? *Nat Rev Rheumatol*. Jun 2016;12(6):367-72. doi:10.1038/nrrheum.2016.18

[107] Lazarus MN, Turner-Stokes T, Chavele KM, Isenberg DA, Ehrenstein MR. B-cell numbers and phenotype at clinical relapse following rituximab therapy differ in SLE patients according to anti-dsDNA antibody levels. *Rheumatology (Oxford)*. Jul 2012;51(7):1208-15. doi:10.1093/rheumatology/ker526

[108] Carter LM, Isenberg DA, Ehrenstein MR. Elevated serum BAFF levels are associated with rising anti-double-stranded DNA antibody levels and disease flare following B cell depletion therapy in systemic lupus erythematosus. *Arthritis Rheum*. Oct 2013;65(10):2672-9. doi:10.1002/art.38074

[109] Díaz-Lagares C, Croca S, Sangle S, et al. Efficacy of rituximab in 164 patients with biopsy-proven lupus nephritis: pooled data from European cohorts. *Autoimmun Rev*. Mar 2012;11(5):357-64. doi:10.1016/j.autrev.2011.10.009

[110] Gomez Mendez LM, Cascino MD, Garg J, et al. Peripheral Blood B Cell Depletion after Rituximab and Complete Response in Lupus Nephritis. *Clin J Am Soc Nephrol*. Oct 8 2018;13(10):1502-1509. doi:10.2215/cjn.01070118

[111] Stohl W. Future prospects in biologic therapy for systemic lupus erythematosus. *Nat Rev Rheumatol*. Dec 2013;9(12):705-20. doi:10.1038/nrrheum.2013.136

[112] Morais SA, Vilas-Boas A, Isenberg DA. B-cell survival factors in autoimmune rheumatic disorders. *Ther Adv Musculoskelet Dis*. Aug 2015;7(4):122-51. doi:10.1177/1759720x15586782

[113] Vilas-Boas A, Morais SA, Isenberg DA. Belimumab in systemic lupus erythematosus. *RMD Open*. 2015;1(1):e000011. doi:10.1136/rmdopen-2014-000011

[114] Naradikian MS, Perate AR, Cancro MP. BAFF receptors and ligands create independent homeostatic niches for B cell subsets. *Curr Opin Immunol*. Jun 2015;34:126-9. doi:10.1016/j.coi.2015.03.005

[115] Vincent FB, Morand EF, Schneider P, Mackay F. The BAFF/APRIL system in SLE pathogenesis. *Nat Rev Rheumatol*. Jun 2014;10(6):365-73. doi:10.1038/nrrheum.2014.33

[116] Dillon SR, Harder B, Lewis KB, et al. B-lymphocyte stimulator/a proliferation-inducing ligand heterotrimers are elevated in the sera of patients with autoimmune disease and are neutralized by atacicept and B-cell maturation antigen-immunoglobulin. *Arthritis Res Ther*. 2010;12(2):R48. doi:10.1186/ar2959

[117] Roschke V, Sosnovtseva S, Ward CD, et al. BLyS and APRIL form biologically active heterotrimers that are expressed in patients with systemic immune-based rheumatic diseases. *J Immunol*. Oct 15 2002;169(8):4314-21. doi:10.4049/jimmunol.169.8.4314

[118] Stohl W. Systemic lupus erythematosus and its ABCs (APRIL/

BLyS complexes). *Arthritis Res Ther*. 2010:111. vol. 2.

[119] Mok MY. The immunological basis of B-cell therapy in systemic lupus erythematosus. *Int J Rheum Dis*. Feb 1 2010;13(1):3-11. doi:10.1111/j.1756-185X.2009.01458.x

[120] Batten M, Groom J, Cachero TG, et al. BAFF mediates survival of peripheral immature B lymphocytes. *J Exp Med*. Nov 20 2000;192(10):1453-66. doi:10.1084/jem.192.10.1453

[121] Mackay F, Schneider P, Rennert P, Browning J. BAFF AND APRIL: a tutorial on B cell survival. *Annu Rev Immunol*. 2003;21:231-64. doi:10.1146/annurev.immunol.21.120601.141152

[122] Guerreiro Castro S, Isenberg DA. Belimumab in systemic lupus erythematosus (SLE): evidence-to-date and clinical usefulness. *Ther Adv Musculoskelet Dis*. Mar 2017;9(3):75-85. doi:10.1177/1759720x17690474

[123] Jones A, Muller P, Dore CJ, et al. Belimumab after B cell depletion therapy in patients with systemic lupus erythematosus (BEAT Lupus) protocol: a prospective multicentre, double-blind, randomised, placebo-controlled, 52-week phase II clinical trial. *BMJ Open*. Dec 16 2019;9(12):e032569. doi:10.1136/bmjopen-2019-032569

[124] Plüß M, Tampe B, Niebusch N, Zeisberg M, Müller GA, Korsten P. Clinical Efficacy of Routinely Administered Belimumab on Proteinuria and Neuropsychiatric Lupus. *Front Med (Lausanne)*. 2020;7:222. doi:10.3389/fmed.2020.00222

[125] Furie R, Rovin BH, Houssiau F, et al. Two-Year, Randomized, Controlled Trial of Belimumab in Lupus Nephritis. *N Engl J Med*. Sep 17 2020;383(12):1117-1128. doi:10.1056/NEJMoa2001180

[126] Reddy V, Klein C, Isenberg DA, et al. Obinutuzumab induces superior B-cell cytotoxicity to rituximab in rheumatoid arthritis and systemic lupus erythematosus patient samples. *Rheumatology (Oxford)*. Jul 1 2017;56(7):1227-1237. doi:10.1093/rheumatology/kex067

[127] Reddy V, Dahal LN, Cragg MS, Leandro M. Optimising B-cell depletion in autoimmune disease: is obinutuzumab the answer? *Drug Discov Today*. Aug 2016;21(8):1330-8. doi:10.1016/j.drudis.2016.06.009

[128] Hassan SU, Md Yusof MY, Emery P, Dass S, Vital EM. Biologic Sequencing in Systemic Lupus Erythematosus: After Secondary Non-response to Rituximab, Switching to Humanised Anti-CD20 Agent Is More Effective Than Belimumab. *Front Med (Lausanne)*. 2020;7:498. doi:10.3389/fmed.2020.00498

[129] Sanford M, McCormack PL. Ofatumumab. *Drugs*. May 28 2010;70(8):1013-9. doi:10.2165/11203850-000000000-00000

[130] Speth F, Hinze C, Häfner R. Combination of ofatumumab and fresh frozen plasma in hypocomplementemic systemic lupus erythematosus: a case report. *Lupus*. Jul 2018;27(8):1395-1396. doi:10.1177/0961203318756289

[131] Masoud S, McAdoo SP, Bedi R, Cairns TD, Lightstone L. Ofatumumab for B cell depletion in patients with systemic lupus erythematosus who are allergic to rituximab. *Rheumatology (Oxford)*. Jul 1 2018;57(7):1156-1161. doi:10.1093/rheumatology/key042

[132] Rao V, Gordon C. Evaluation of epratuzumab as a biologic therapy in systemic lupus erythematosus. *Immunotherapy*. 2014;6(11):1165-75. doi:10.2217/imt.14.80

[133] Geh D, Gordon C. Epratuzumab for the treatment of systemic lupus erythematosus. *Expert Rev Clin Immunol*. Apr 2018;14(4):245-258. doi:10.1080/1744666x.2018.1450141

[134] Gottenberg JE, Dörner T, Bootsma H, et al. Efficacy of Epratuzumab, an Anti-CD22 Monoclonal IgG Antibody, in Systemic Lupus Erythematosus Patients With Associated Sjögren's Syndrome: Post Hoc Analyses From the EMBODY Trials. *Arthritis Rheumatol*. May 2018;70(5):763-773. doi:10.1002/art.40425

[135] Schneider WM, Chevillotte MD, Rice CM. Interferon-stimulated genes: a complex web of host defenses. *Annu Rev Immunol*. 2014;32:513-45. doi:10.1146/annurev-immunol-032713-120231

[136] Rönnblom L. The importance of the type I interferon system in autoimmunity. *Clin Exp Rheumatol*. Jul-Aug 2016;34(4 Suppl 98):21-4.

[137] Khamashta M, Merrill JT, Werth VP, et al. Sifalimumab, an anti-interferon-α monoclonal antibody, in moderate to severe systemic lupus erythematosus: a randomised, double-blind, placebo-controlled study. *Ann Rheum Dis*. Nov 2016;75(11):1909-1916. doi:10.1136/annrheumdis-2015-208562

[138] Zimmer R, Scherbarth HR, Rillo OL, Gomez-Reino JJ, Muller S. Lupuzor/P140 peptide in patients with systemic lupus erythematosus: a randomised, double-blind, placebo-controlled phase IIb clinical trial. *Ann Rheum Dis*. Nov 2013;72(11):1830-5. doi:10.1136/annrheumdis-2012-202460

[139] Rutkowski K, Sowa P, Rutkowska-Talipska J, Kuryliszyn-Moskal A, Rutkowski R. Dehydroepiandrosterone (DHEA): hypes and hopes. *Drugs*. Jul 2014;74(11):1195-207. doi:10.1007/s40265-014-0259-8

[140] Petri MA, Lahita RG, Van Vollenhoven RF, et al. Effects of prasterone on corticosteroid requirements of women with systemic lupus erythematosus: a double-blind, randomized, placebo-controlled trial. *Arthritis Rheum*. Jul 2002;46(7):1820-9. doi:10.1002/art.10364

[141] Sánchez-Guerrero J, Fragoso-Loyo HE, Neuwelt CM, et al. Effects of prasterone on bone mineral density in women with active systemic lupus erythematosus receiving chronic glucocorticoid therapy. *J Rheumatol*. Aug 2008;35(8):1567-75.

[142] Targher G, Pichiri I, Lippi G. Vitamin D, thrombosis, and hemostasis: more than skin deep. *Semin Thromb Hemost*. Feb 2012;38(1):114-24. doi:10.1055/s-0031-1300957

[143] Brøndum-Jacobsen P, Benn M, Tybjaerg-Hansen A, Nordestgaard BG. 25-Hydroxyvitamin D concentrations and risk of venous thromboembolism in the general population with 18,791 participants. *J Thromb Haemost*. Mar 2013;11(3):423-31. doi:10.1111/jth.12118

[144] Petri M, Bello KJ, Fang H, Magder LS. Vitamin D in systemic lupus erythematosus: modest association with disease activity and the urine protein-to-creatinine ratio. *Arthritis Rheum*. Jul 2013;65(7):1865-71. doi:10.1002/art.37953

[145] Andreoli L, Dall'Ara F, Piantoni S, et al. A 24-month prospective study on the efficacy and safety of two different monthly regimens of vitamin D supplementation in pre-menopausal women with systemic lupus erythematosus. *Lupus*. Apr 2015;24(4-5):499-506. doi:10.1177/0961203314559089

[146] Aranow C, Kamen DL, Dall'Era M, et al. Randomized, Double-Blind, Placebo-Controlled Trial of the Effect of Vitamin D3 on the Interferon Signature in Patients With Systemic Lupus Erythematosus. *Arthritis Rheumatol*. Jul 2015;67(7):1848-57. doi:10.1002/art.39108

[147] van Vollenhoven RF, Mosca M, Bertsias G, et al. Treat-to-target in systemic lupus erythematosus: recommendations from an international task force. *Ann Rheum Dis*. Jun 2014;73(6):958-67. doi:10.1136/annrheumdis-2013-205139

[148] Fanouriakis A, Kostopoulou M, Alunno A, et al. 2019 update of the EULAR recommendations for the management of systemic lupus erythematosus. *Ann Rheum Dis*. Jun 2019;78(6):736-745. doi:10.1136/annrheumdis-2019-215089

[149] Furie R, Khamashta M, Merrill JT, et al. Anifrolumab, an Anti-Interferon-α Receptor Monoclonal Antibody, in Moderate-to-Severe Systemic Lupus Erythematosus. *Arthritis Rheumatol*. Feb 2017;69(2):376-386. doi:10.1002/art.39962

[150] Merrill JT, Furie R, Werth VP, et al. Anifrolumab effects on rash and arthritis: impact of the type I interferon gene signature in the phase IIb MUSE study in patients with systemic lupus erythematosus. *Lupus Sci Med*. 2018;5(1):e000284. doi:10.1136/lupus-2018-000284

[151] Lateef A, Petri M. Biologics in the treatment of systemic lupus erythematosus. *Curr Opin Rheumatol*. Sep 2010;22(5):504-9. doi:10.1097/BOR.0b013e32833b475e

[152] Wallace DJ, Furie RA, Tanaka Y, et al. Baricitinib for systemic lupus erythematosus: a double-blind, randomised, placebo-controlled, phase 2 trial. *Lancet*. Jul 21 2018;392(10143):222-231. doi:10.1016/s0140-6736(18)31363-1

Chapter 7

Clinical Use of Mesenchymal Stem Cells in Treatment of Systemic Lupus Erythematosus

Hulya Bukulmez and Gurinder Kumar

Abstract

Systemic lupus erythematosus (SLE) is a chronic multisystem autoimmune inflammatory disorder with considerable clinical heterogeneity and a prevalence of 26 to 52 out of 100,000. In autoimmune diseases, such as SLE, the immune system loses its ability to distinguish between self and other. Treatment of SLE is challenging because of clinical heterogeneity and unpredictable disease flares. Currently available treatments, such as corticosteroids, cyclophosphamide (CYC), and other immunosuppressive or immunomodulating agents, can control most lupus flares but a definitive cure is rarely achieved. Moreover, standard therapies are associated with severe side effects, including susceptibility to infections, ovarian failure, and secondary malignancy. Alternative therapeutic options that are more efficacious with fewer side effects are needed to improve long-term outcome. Mesenchymal stem cells/multipotent stromal cells (MSCs), which secrete immunomodulatory factors that help restore immune balance, could hold promise for treating these diseases. Because MSCs do not express major histocompatibility complex II (MHC-II) or costimulatory molecules, they are also "immunologically privileged" and less likely to be rejected after transplant. Stem cells are defined as a class of undifferentiated cells in multicellular organisms that are pluripotent and self-replicating. MSCs are promising in regenerative medicine and cell-based therapies due to their abilities of their self-renewal and multilineage differentiation potential. Most importantly, MSCs have immunoregulatory effects on multiple immune system cells. While some studies report safety and efficacy of allogeneic bone marrow and/or umbilical cord MSC transplantation (MSCT) in patients with severe and drug-refractory systemic lupus erythematosus (SLE), others found no apparent additional effect over and above standard immunosuppression. The purpose of this chapter is to discuss immune modulation effects of MSCs and the efficacy of MSCs treatments in SLE.

Keywords: Mesenchymal stem cell, Cell therapy, Systemic Lupus Erythematosus, Clinical trials, Lupus nephritis

1. Introduction

Systemic Lupus Erythematosus (SLE) is a chronic multi system autoimmune inflammatory disease in which vascular inflammation cause devastating organ damage such as end-stage renal disease (ESRD). Sizeable patient populations;

12,600 end-stage kidney disease (ESKD) caused by SLE, are refractory for all current standard of care [1].

Clinical presentations of SLE, prototype autoimmune disease for interferon activation, are highly heterogeneous, ranging from mild systemic inflammation that affects skin or joints to severe organ damage (brain, kidney, lung etc.). Heterogeneity of clinical presentations requires diverse treatment protocols, addressing multiple immune abnormalities affecting variety of organs. The exact etiology of SLE is not completely understood. Pathogenesis of SLE comprises genetic, environmental, and hormonal factors which induces multiple immune cell lines and systems act abnormally which are mostly explained by autoimmune activation. All etiopathogenic immune pathways targeted with chemotherapy or biologics to date have failed to improve some portion of SLE patients. Heterogeneity of clinical presentations require diverse treatment protocols, addressing immune abnormalities.

There is an urgent clinical need for an effective treatment of chronic autoimmune diseases induced by abnormal activation of immune system that result in multiple organ damage in SLE and in others [1–3]. The current standard of care includes high dose corticosteroids, chemotheraphy with azathioprine, cyclophosphamide, mycophenolate mofetil, cyclosporin, and combination of all with biologics such as rituximab (Anti-CD20) or belimumab (anti-Blsy) [4, 5]. Current modalities that are available to treat SLE and SLE like diseases are immune suppressive and have toxic side effects. After treatments with corticosteroids and chemotherapy, patients become even more vulnerable to pathogens and develop sepsis and septic shock. In many patients, even combinations of all available medications are not effective in controlling the disease progression and development of end stage organ failure. Innovation of nontoxic cellular therapies that target both, the vascular wall and the immune responses within the local microenvironment, are needed.

In many patients, even combinations of all available medications are not effective in controlling the disease progression and development of end stage organ failure. Collectively, at least 10–15% of patients fail to respond to all existing treatments. Specifically, three groups of SLE patients with the greatest unmet need include:

1. 7–8% of patients who have severe nervous system involvement refractory to cytotoxic and immune suppressing medications [6];

2. 10–30% patients with severe nephritis who do not respond to cytotoxic and immune suppressing therapy or available biologic treatment (such as belimumab and rituximab) and become dependent on dialysis leading to death within 15 years [1]; and

3. 2–5% of patients develop thrombotic thrombocytopenic purpura who do not respond to combination of cytotoxic medications, immune suppressants, plasma exchange, and biologics, with mortality rate of 34–62% [7].

Disease burden of SLE and lupus nephritis in the US is estimated at 313,436 (100/100,000) and 63,256 (20/100,000), respectively [8–10]. Approximately 10 to 20 percent of patients with lupus nephritis progress to end-stage renal disease as they do not respond to commercially available treatments.

Unfortunately, there is still no uniformly effective treatment targeting both cellular and humoral autoimmunity for SLE. Therapies targeting components of cellular or humoral immune system fails to induce sustained remission in disease activity in multicenter clinical trials. To design a new treatment that can control the cellular and innate immune activation and regenerate the damaged organs in active SLE, the understanding of the degree and exact kind of the immune dysregulation is necessary. Multiple immune cells and immune signaling pathways have been studied in etiopathogenesis of SLE and have been found to act abnormally. While a set of cells clonally expand and act abnormally, we see some of the cells that have homeostatic roles in controlling self-tolerance are diminished or dysfunctional in SLE.

2. Immune dysregulation that leads to SLE

Pathogenesis of SLE comprises genetic, environmental, and hormonal factors resulting in multi-system autoimmune inflammatory disease. **Systemic Lupus Erythematosus** [11] is suggested to be the prototype of several systemic inflammatory diseases that are induced by abnormal activation of the type I (−α, −β) [12] and II (−ɣ) interferon (IFN) [13] pathways. Interferon activation results in multiple immune cellular abnormalities, including; dendritic cells (DC), natural killer (NK) cells, cytotoxic T cells, T regulatory cells (Tregs), and autoreactive B cells [14].

SLE is characterized by irregularities in innate cellular and humoral immunity functions [15]. Abnormal T-cells and B-cells recognize self-antigens resulting in immune hyperactivity and autoantibody production that ends up in a multisystem inflammatory disease.

Immune dysregulation in SLE has been described by not one but multiple cell lineages such as CD4+ and CD8+ T-cells, dendritic cells (DC), Natural Killer (NK) cells, B-cell overproduction of autoantibodies, and T regulatory (Treg) cell dysfunction. CD8+ T cells and NK cells have decreased cytotoxic activity. There is a general inability of TGF- β production, which in return accounts for sustained T and B cell hyperactivity and reduced Tregs activity and numbers. There is a disproportional balance between the activated and tolerogenic DCs during SLE activity that limits the expansion of Tregs [16]. The remaining small amount of Tregs that are still existing during the inflammatory activity of lupus are not sufficient to overcome the strong T-cell activation [17, 18].

In both human patients with SLE and in lupus prone mice models, CD4 + CD25 + Foxp3+ Tregs are reported to be decreased during disease activity. CD4+ T helper cell subset (Th17 cells) are increased in SLE in response to IL-17 activation [19, 20]. Blockage of IL-17 has also been suggested as a new treatment option [21, 22].

Restoration of T-cell functions are important for disease control. On the other hand, lupus-like autoimmunity can result simply due to B-cell hyperactivity, with either minimal or no contribution from T-lymphocytes. B cell hyperactivity results with production variety of IgG and IgM autoantibodies directed against nuclear components such as double stranded (ds) DNA and/or single stranded (ss) DNA. Both anti-ssDNA and anti-dsDNA are involved in disease pathogenesis and clinical progress [23, 24].

The type I interferon system appears to play a critical role in SLE etiopathology [11, 25–27]. All the cellular and humoral immune abnormalities seem to activate type I interferons, which in return charge the immune cells further and result in loss of tolerance. Type I interferons control dendritic cell maturation into antigen presenting cells which contribute to B-cell hyperactivity and induce a Th1 response and sustain T-cell activation [28, 29]. Type I interferons are not controlled well and are in excess amount partially due to deficiency of Treg activities in SLE [30–33].

Another major etiopathogenic immune pathway is explained by multiple complement pathway abnormalities. Complement deficiency can be seen up to 5% of all lupus patients [34]. In addition, 50% of SLE patients with deficiencies or dysfunction of the early classical complement pathway develop a lupus-like disease.

3. MSC treatment in SLE

While there is systemic inflammation and autoimmunity ongoing, patients with SLE have less active immune cells that defend against pathogens and tumors [35, 36]. Cytotoxic CD8+ T cells and T regulatory (Treg) cells that play fundamental role in immune defense are depleted during SLE activity [37].

Currently available treatments of SLE (Systemic Lupus Erythematosus) target one cell (CD20+ B cells) or one pathway at a time leaving the others to continue to function abnormally and their immunosuppressant side effects to diminish patients' ability to fight infections. After these treatments, patients become immune compromised and vulnerable to pathogens and develop sepsis and septic shock. In many patients, even combinations of all are not effective in controlling disease progression sometimes developing end stage organ failure.

MSCs are multipotent stromal cells than have the potential to differentiate into multiple mesenchymal lineages [38–43]. Core standardized definition of the 'multipotent mesenchymal stromal cell' as a plastic-adherent cell type bearing various stromal surface makers, but lacking hematopoietic markers, capable of at least osteogenic, chondrogenic and adipogenic differentiation was proposed by a consensus group [44]. The name was later modified and was changed to 'mesenchymal stromal cell'. No unique marker exists to define MSCs still and clinical studies will certainly involve different heterogeneous MSCs that can be isolated from different adult and fetal tissues such bone marrow (BM), umbilical cord (UC) and adipose tissue (AT). MSCs are so far defined with the presence of their characteristic cell surface markers such as CD105, CD90, CD73, CD106, CD146, CD166, CD271 and the absence of hematopoietic progenitor cells markers such as CD45, CD34 and CD14. They are uniquely immune privileged and can escape rejection reactions from hosts since they do not express class II MHC, such as HLA-DR and co-stimulatory molecules such as CD80, CD86 and CD40 [43, 45, 46]. Therefore, they are easily used as adoptive transfer cell treatment without any prior immune ablation therapies.

Besides their differentiation potentials, MSCs have potent immune regulatory effects. MSCs mediate immune system either by secreting soluble factors or directly interacting with a variety of immune effector cells. MSCs uniquely gain different properties and immunoregulatory effects depending on the inflammatory milieu and disease setting. MSCs secrete numerous cytokines, chemokines, and hormones to exert paracrine effects on adjacent immune cells to modulate their proliferation, differentiation, migration, and adhesion functions under injury conditions.

It has been suggested that with their potent immune regulatory effects MSCs are future of cell therapy in refractory lupus. However, the studies thus far published do not agree on the kind, amount and frequency of MSC treatments or showed consistent efficacy. MSCs have not been FDA approved for any disease indication, mostly due to challenges in potency. MSCs have been used as therapeutics in hundreds of clinical trials, including SLE, with no adverse reactions reported.

4. Immune modulating effects of MSCs that may help suppressing auto inflammatory activity during SLE

MSCs produce a collection of immune modulating molecules, which can locally (paracrine) or systemically (endocrine) effect inflammation. The actions of MSCs are dependent on the environmental signals they receive and are directed to control the excess inflammatory response. It is well studies that MSCs can switch the T cell balance from a pro-inflammatory Th1 phenotype (secreting INF-γ and TNF-α) or Th17 phenotype (secreting IL-17) [47] to an anti-inflammatory to Th2 profile (secreting IL-4) (**Figure 1**) [48, 49].

More relevant MSC activities that may help in SLE treatment are 1) MSCs decrease IFN-γ production *in vitro* by T-cells [50] 2) MSCs are able to modulate the cytokine-production profile of (*in vivo*) differentiated Th17 cells, as well as the production of the IL-17 [51–53], 3) MSCs also influence the development and function of DCs [54, 55], 4) MSCs promote the generation of antigen-specific Tregs either directly or indirectly by modulating dendritic cells (DCs) [56], 5) MSCs modulate macrophages [57–60] 6) down-regulate the production of pro-inflammatory cytokines TNF-α, IL-1, IL-6 and IL-12p70 and increase the production of anti-inflammatory cytokine IL-10, 7) enhance the phagocytic activity which in return induce resolution of inflammation [61–63] (**Figure 1**).

MSCs can suppress proliferation of both CD4+ and CD8+ T lymphocytes in vitro in a dose-dependent, non-apoptotic-induced manner, and the immunosuppressive properties against T cells varies among different MSC sources. Transforming growth factor-β (TGF-β), prostaglandin E2 (PGE2), nitric oxide (NO), and indoleamine 2,3-dioxygenase (IDO) have been reported to be involved in the MSC-mediated T cell suppression. CD8+ T cells and their activation axis with Indolamine 2, 3-Dioxygenase (IDO) an important anti-inflammatory factor, is suggested to be required for successful suppression of SLE [64], and there is significant data showing the need to increase the Treg activity in SLE treatment (**Figure 1**) [51].

One key element of the possible effect of MSCs in SLE is that once MSCs enter the inflammatory environment particularly those SLE affected or injured organs;

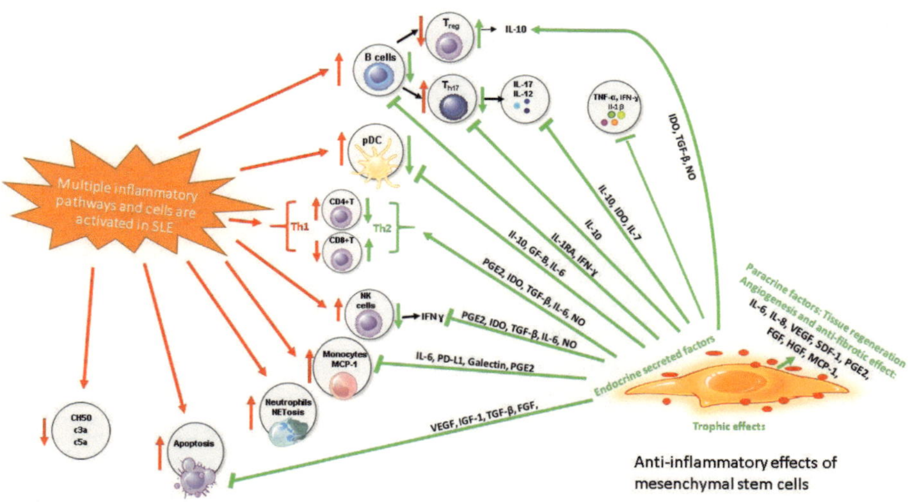

Figure 1.
Suggested pathways of how anti-inflammatory effects of MSCs that control the loss of tolerance, cellular dysfunction and inflammation. During SLE active disease multiple immune cells that works in both innate and adaptive immune system are dysfunctional leading to loss of tolerance and sever inflammation. MSCs, can sense the inflammatory microenvironment and act on attenuating inflammatory activity by secreting soluble factors, such as IDO, TGF-β, PGE-2. VEGF, BMP-7, TNF-α, IL-6, IL-7and IL-10, i.e. endocrine effect. MSC exert the immunomodulatory function by promoting a switch from pro-inflammatory to anti-inflammatory phenotype and cytokine secretion by T- cells, dendritic cells and NK cells. MSCs can inhibit the proliferation and activation of B effector cells and CD4 + T lymphocytes, while changing and strengthening the cytotoxic effects of CD8 + T cells and NK cells. MSCs anti-inflammatory effects is also explained by its effect on increase of the Tregs, while its potent effect in decreasing the IL-17 secreting Th17 cells. Red arrows are showing the SLE inflammation activation signaling for pathogenic cellular expansion or decrease, while green arrows and blunted lines are showing the opposing effects of MSCs on the abnormal cellular activation and anti-inflammatory effects. MSCs endocrine secreted factors by which they are suggested to act specific cellular expansion and activity are defined on the arrows.

their immune-modulatory phenotype could become activated by IFN-γ, TNF-α and IL-1β in the microenvironment [65]. Furthermore, it has been shown that MSCs are chemotactically drawn toward a variety of wound healing cytokines in vitro, including IL-1 and TNF-α. These data suggest that MSCs or endogenous cells resembling MSCs, such as pericytes, are likely to migrate to and participate in the response to tissue injury [66–69].

When MSCs are exposed to the microenvironment of diseased tissue, they control/suppress inflammation inducing regeneration [56]. With their potent immune regulatory and regenerative effects in response to their microenvironment, and as no adverse reactions in clinical trials have been reported, MSCs are an attractive treatment in SLE. By increasing the potency of MSCs in SLE, it is anticipated that primed MSCs will lower the overall cost of care for SLE patients that are refractory for the current standard of care.

Effects of human MSCs on interferon regulated mediators, and the connections of these mediators with clinical outcomes in SLE have been suggested, but MSC treatments have not been efficacious across heterogeneous organ involvement of SLE to date.

MSCs have been used as therapeutics in hundreds of clinical trials, as of July 2020, there were a total of 1,138 registered clinical trials to clinicaltrials.gov including SLE. In the 18 published clinical trials with outcomes there were no serious adverse events reported [70]. However, MSCs have not been FDA approved for any disease indication yet, mostly due to challenges in potency. MSC treatment has been shown to be successful for a short time and there were relapses in SLE patients in 6–12 months [71, 72].

MSC sources used in clinical trials have different donor pools and are isolated from different tissues with variable immune regulatory function. Furthermore, large-scale MSC-based cell therapy remains restricted due to the cells' ability to expand, and then efficiently respond to inflammatory environment after several number of passages.

5. Recent SLE clinical trials using stem cells

Stem cell treatment to those SLE patients who have been refractory to all known therapies have been the last resort. Although the results of studies reported in early 2000 suggested that autologous stem cells treatment (ASCT) suggested the efficacy for remission induction of refractory SLE, mortality among those patients with longer disease duration was particularly high and mostly due to immune suppressive procedure (12%). Almost 30 percent patients relapsed after therapy and longer duration of immune suppressive therapies post ASCT was suggested [73, 74]. It was clearly shown that severe myeloablative therapies prior to ASCT's to SLE patients who already have immune compromised status the success rate has been poor. Therefore, other groups assessed the safety of intense immunosuppression and autologous hematopoietic stem cell support in patients with severe and treatment refractory SLE [75, 76]. Overall 5-year survival of those SLE patients was 84%, and probability of disease-free survival at 5 years following HSCT was 50% (**Table 1**).

While the initial stem cell clinical trials were being performed for treatment of SLE, first report of successful MSC treatment in a child with acute graft-versus-host disease (GvHD) using allogeneic MSCs was published in 2004 [89]. After two infusions of bone-marrow-derived MSCs obtained from his mother this child responded very well to the infusion treatment. Following the success of this pediatric case with GVHD, multiple preclinical animal studies and other human clinical trials for treatment of other autoimmune diseases started to take place. The initial

Reference (First author, date)	Study type/ SLE, organ involvement	Number of patients studied, Age range	MSC source*	Type and amount (dose)	Prior treatment	Outcome criteria	Improvement (%) in 6 months	Improvement (%) in 12 m and above
Jayne et al. (2004) [74]	Retrospective registry. SLE or nephritis	53, (9–52 yo)	Peripheral blood (n = 44), bone marrow (n = 8), from both (n = 1)	Autologous stem cell treatment (ASCT)	Cyclophosphamide (84%), anti-thymocyte globulin (76%) and lymphoid irradiation (22%)	SLEDAI, brain MR scan, pulmonary function tests, echocardiogram, serum creatinine, ANA, anti-dsDNA, other anti-nuclear autoantibodies and C3, C4	Remission rate (based on a reduction of the SLEDAI to <3) in 66%, one-third of whom later relapsed to some degree.	Mortality 12% at one year
Burt et al. (2006) [75]	Single arm trial. Severe fractory SLE	50, Mean age (SD) 30(10.9) years	Peripheral blood	Autologous stem cell treatment (ASCT)	IV Cyc, 50 mg/kg daily, before transplantation (total dose 200 mg/kg) and intravenous equine ATG, 30 mg/kg daily, before transplantation (total dose 90 mg/kg).	Primary, survival, disease-free. Secondary end points included (SLEDAI), ANA and anti– (ds) DNA, C3 and C4, and changes in renal and pulmonary organ function assessed before treatment and at 6 months, 12 months, and then yearly for 5 years.	2/50 patients died after mobilization 48 patients underwent HSCT. Treatment-related mortality was 2% (1/50). By intention to treat, treatment-related mortality was 4% (2/50). Renal function stabilized and improved SLEDAI, ANA, anti-ds DNA, complement, and carbon monoxide diffusion lung capacity adjusted for hemoglobin.	5-year survival was 84% and probability of disease-free survival at 5 years following HSCT was 50%.

Reference (First author, date)	Study type/ SLE, organ involvement	Number of patients studied, Age range	MSC source*	Type and amount (dose)	Prior treatment	Outcome criteria	Improvement (%) in 6 months	Improvement (%) in 12 m and above
Sun et al. (2010) [77]	Single arm SLE nephritis	16	UC MSC	Allogeneic	Cyclophosphamide iv for 2–4 days	Percent Tregs improved in 3 months		Decreased SLEDAI and proteinuria in all patients in 28 months
Liang et al. (2010) [78]	Single arm SLE nephritis	15				Percentage of Treg cells increased at 1 week and 3 and 6 months ($P < 0.05$)		Decreased SLEDAI and proteinuria in all patients
Carrion F et al. (2010) [79]	SLE	2 (19 yr., 25 yr)	BM-derived MSCs,	Autologous, 1×10^6/kg			Disease activity indexes and immunological parameters were assessed at baseline, 1, 2, 7 and 14 weeks	
Shi D et al. (2012) [80]	SLE associated diffuse alveolar hemorrhage.	4 (32 ± 15 years)	UC-MSCT	Allogenic	1×10^6/kg	hemoglobin, platelet level, oxygen saturation, and serological factors. High-resolution CT (HRCT) scans of the chest were performed to evaluate pulmonary manifestation	Clinical changes before and after transplantation	

Reference (First author, date)	Study type/ SLE, organ involvement	Number of patients studied, Age range	MSC source*	Type and amount (dose)	Prior treatment	Outcome criteria	Improvement (%) in 6 months	Improvement (%) in 12 m and above
Wang et al. (2012) [81]	Unblinded, randomized, 2-arm/12 months	58	BM/UC MSC single vs. 2× every 7 days		CYC 10 mg/kg per day, day 4, 3, and 2			Complete remission 1× 53% 2× 29%
X Li et al. (2013) [82]	SLE refractory cytopenia	35(16–62 years)	BM/UC MSC.	Allogenic 1×10^6/kg	1 = Pretreatment group: (15/35) Cyc 0.4–1.8 gm IV for 2–4 days 2 = No Cyc Pretreatment (20/35)	CBC's Hb and Platelet, Th17, Treg, SLEDAI	57% patients with leukopenia and 68% patients with thrombocytopenia showed hematological improvement.	75% of SLE remained stable after 12 months
Wang et al. (2013) [83]	Severe and refractory SLE	87(12–56 years)	BM/ UC-MSC	Allogenic 1×10^6/kg	Pretreatment 59% Cyc 10 mg/kg/day IV on day −4, −3, −2. 36% No treatment	Primary: Survival, disease remission and relapse, transplantation-related adverse events. Secondary: SLEDAI and serology	Complete clinical remission 28% at 1 year Relapse rates 12% at 1 year.	Complete clinical remission rate was 31% at 2 years (12/39), 42% at 3 years (5/12), and 50% at 4 years (3/6). 4-year follow-up overall rate of survival was 94% (82/87).
				One-time treatment				

Reference (First author, date)	Study type/ SLE, organ involvement	Number of patients studied, Age range	MSC source*	Type and amount (dose)	Prior treatment	Outcome criteria	Improvement (%) in 6 months	Improvement (%) in 12 m and above
Fei Gu et al. (2014) [72]	Open Label and single center Active and refractory Lupus Nephritis	81(12–55 years)	BM or UC-derived MSC	Allogenic 1×10^6/kg	No IV Cyc pretreatment. vs. Pretransplant medication: Pred/ Cyclophosphamide(monthly)/ MMF	Primary outcome: Renal remission (complete/ partial) as well as renal flares. The secondary outcome included renal activity score	The mean leukocyte counts still stayed normal for 5 patients completing 24-month follow-up	For 24 SLE patients with anemia, normalized remained stable at 12- and 24-month visits
Wang et al. (2014) [71]	Severe and refractory SLE	40, (17–54 years)	UC-MSC	Allogenic	No IV Cyc pretreatment. 26/40 pts. received Cyc as a basal treatment.	Safety, Major clinical response (MCR), Partial clinical response (PCR) and relapse. SLEDAI, BILAG and renal functional indices	Disease relapse at 9 months 12.5%, at 12 months 16.7% of follow-up.	Survival rate was 92.5% in 12 months.
				1×10^6/kg at 0 and 7 days				
							32.5% achieved MCR and 27.5% achieved PCR, during 12 months.	

Reference (First author, date)	Study type/ SLE, organ involvement	Number of patients studied, Age range	MSC source*	Type and amount (dose)	Prior treatment	Outcome criteria	Improvement (%) in 6 months	Improvement (%) in 12 m and above
Deng et al. (2017) [84]	Randomized, double blind, placebo controlled SLE nephritis	18 patients Randomized. 12 patients h UC-MSC group and 6 patients placebo group. Mean age in both groups 29 years.	UC-MSC	Allogenic	11/18 pts. received methylprednisolone and CYP induction therapy, and the 12th to 18th patients enrolled received IV. methylprednisolone only and intravenous CYP	24 h urine protein, serum albumin, serum creatinine, SLEDAI and BILAG scores, C3, C4, anti-dsDNA and ANA	Remission occurred in 75% in the hUC-MSC group and 83% in the placebo group.	Stopped in less than 12 months due to lack of efficacy
				20×10^6/ patient one time				
Chen C et al. (2017) [85]	Active SLE refractory to conventional treatment	10	UC-MSCT	1×10^6/kg		Soluble human leukocyte antigen G was measured 24 h and 1 mo after infusion	Negative correlation between s HLA-G levels and SLEDAI score.	
Wang et al. (2018) [86]	Open-label phase II Severe and drug refractory SLE	81(12–62 years)	BM or UC-MSC	Allogeneic 1×10^6/kg (Multiple infusions of MSCs were permitted)	39/81 received IV Cyc (10 mg/kg/day) in days −4, −3, −2; 42/81- no IV Cyc.	5-year overall survival. Complete and partial clinical remission.		5-year overall survival rate was 84%.
					Patients receiving repeat MSCT, no IV Cyc used.			

Reference (First author, date)	Study type/ SLE, organ involvement	Number of patients studied, Age range	MSC source*	Type and amount (dose)	Prior treatment	Outcome criteria	Improvement (%) in 6 months	Improvement (%) in 12 m and above
J Barbado et al. (2018) [87]	Active SLE with proteinuria (1,000 mg in 24 h) and class IV proliferative nephritis	3(40–45years)	BM-MSC	Allogenic 1.5×10^6/kg	Patients were pretreated with variety of chemotherapy before enrollment to the study	The 24-h proteinuria level, glomerular hematuria, leukocyturia, serum creatinine, and the glomerular filtration rate was measured just before treatment (0), and at 1, 3, 6, and 9 months after treatment.	100% of patients showed decreased level of proteinuria SLEDAI scores revealed early, durable, and substantial remissions	Follow up stopped after 9 months
Yuan X et al. (2019) [88]	SLE refractory to conventional therapies	21	UC-MSCT	Allogenic 1×10^6/kg		To study the mechanisms of immunoregulatory mechanism in SLE patients.	Number of peripheral tolerogenic $CD1c^+$ dendritic cells and levels of serum FLT3L are significantly decreased in SLE patients esp. with lupus nephritis compared with healthy controls. Following transplant, significant upregulation of peripheral blood $CD1c^+$ dendritic cells and serum FLT3L was seen.	

Reference (First author, date)	Study type/ SLE, organ involvement	Number of patients studied, Age range	MSC source*	Type and amount (dose)	Prior treatment	Outcome criteria	Improvement (%) in 6 months	Improvement (%) in 12 m and above
Wen L et al. (2019) [88]	Retrospective cohort study SLE pts. with active disease (SLEDAI score > =8	69	BM-/ UC-MSCs	Allogenic 1×10^6/kg		SLE symptoms and SLEDAI scores were assessed at baseline and during follow up to determine low disease activity and clinical remission at 1, 3, 6 and 12 months. To identify predictors of clinical response to allogenic BM or UC MSC treatment		Severe SLE pts. undergo sustained clinical remission with reduced disease maintained over a 1 year follow up. Older age, no arthralgia/ arthritis at baseline, and no prior CYC or HCQ treatment had better first year outcomes after allogenic BM-UC-MSC transplantation.

UC, umbilical cord; bone marrow (BM) or adipogenic (AD) tissue derived MSCs; CYC, cyclophosphamide; HCQ, Hydroxychloroquine.

Table 1.
Human clinical trials that used mesenchymal stem cells (MSCs) for treatment of systemic lupus erythematosus.

approach to MSC treatment took hematopoietic stem cell replacement therapies (HSCT) as examples, and protocols that mimicked HSCT were investigated. One similarity was to use autologous cells rather than allogeneic stem cells and the other similarity was to use myeloablation therapies with chemotherapy agents before the MSC treatment.

While autologous MSC treatment trials showed efficacy in increasing the amount of immune regulatory cells that play an important role in SLE, the clinical disease activity scores were not changed [79]. Same center that published the failure in 2 patients treated with autologous MSCs also performed a study using allogeneic MSCs in 15 patients and showed efficacy [78]. Because sources of allogeneic MSCs are more available and carry less concern of being defective due to disease state or genetic background [90], the following SLE clinical trials used mostly allogeneic MSC sources from variable tissues.

Initial reports of allogeneic MSC trials came from a group of investigators from China. Sun et al. reported a study performed between April 2007 to July 2009 on 16 patients with active SLE nephritis who were enrolled and underwent allogeneic umbilical cord (UC) driven MSC treatment. Study showed efficacy of allogeneic UC MSCs in SLE and suggested that clinical remission was correlating to the increase in peripheral Treg cells and an improved balance between Th1- and Th2- cytokines [77]. Cellular significance was correlating with the decreased amount of proteinuria and decreased SLEDAI (Systemic Lupus Erythematosus Disease Activity Index) scores. Patients in this trial received IV cyclophosphamide treatment for 2–4 days prior to UC MSC treatment.

Same group continued to treat resistant SLE patients and enrolled eighty-seven patients with persistently active SLE who were refractory to standard treatment or had severe organ involvement. While some patients received allogeneic bone marrow some received umbilical cord derived MSCs intravenously (1×10^6 cells/kg of body weight). Three of them were given a second UC-MSC treatment (8, 3, 4 months after the first BM MSC treatment and one was given UC-MSCT additional three times (11, 19, 20 months after the first BM MSC treatment). During the 4-year follow-up the overall rate of survival was 94% (82/87). Complete clinical remission rate was 28% at 1 year (23/83). The overall rate of relapse was 23% (20/87). Only five patients (6%) died after MSC treatment from non-treatment-related events in the 4-year follow-up. Allogeneic MSC were suggested to result in the induction of clinical remission and improvement in organ dysfunction in drug resistant severe SLE patients [83].

Debate of allogeneic versus autologous stem cell treatment continued while initial phase I and II trials were ongoing with MSCs. Sui et al. [91] compared the research of autologous or allogeneic HSC/MSC in SLE. They analyzed the data of Wang et al. [83] i.e. allogeneic group and that of Jayne et al. [74] and Burt et al. [75], i.e. autologous group. In conclusion, they found that the rate of complete clinical remission was similar in these clinical trials (approximately 50%). However, there was higher overall survival rate, lower overall rate of relapse and no transplantation-related mortality in the allogeneic group. Because these 3 studies were not randomized, and it was not possible to compare them with each other exactly due to the heterogeneous disease manifestation at baseline. Authors suggested the importance of randomized clinical trials consisting of a large sample and long term follow up of these patients to further investigate the efficacy and safety of autologous/allogeneic stem cell transplantation [91].

X Li et al. [82, 92] further assessed the roles of allogeneic (BM and UC) MSC treatment with in SLE patients with refractory cytopenia. Thirty-five SLE patients with refractory cytopenia were enrolled and hematological changes of pre- and post-transplantation were evaluated. Significant improvements in blood cell count were found after MSC treatment for most patients, in parallel with the decline of disease activity. Clinical remission was again correlating with increased Treg cells and decreased Th17 cells. Results suggested that MSCs are successful in correcting refractory cytopenia in SLE patients which might be associated with reconstitution of Treg and Th17.

Use of chemotherapy together or before MSC treatment for induction was also assessed by variety of small clinical trials. Wang et al. [71] found no differences between the patient groups that received pretreatment with cyclophosphamide and untreated with cyclophosphamide. There was no difference in the rate of clinical remission after MSC treatments [71]. In addition there were significant number of patients that developed relapse in 6 months and additional MSC treatments were given to those patients with relapse.

Fei Gu et al. [72] assessed the role of allogeneic MSC treatment to induce renal remission in patients with active and refractory lupus nephritis (LN). They conducted an open-label and single-center clinical trial conducted from 2007 to 2010 in which 81 Chinese patients with active and refractory LN were enrolled. Allogeneic bone marrow- or umbilical cord-derived mesenchymal stem cells (MSCs) were administered intravenously at the dose of 1 million cells per kilogram of bodyweight. During the 12-month follow-up, the overall rate of survival was 95% (77/81). Totally, 60.5% (49/81) patients achieved renal remission during 12-month visit by MSCT. Eleven of 49 (22.4%) patients experienced renal flare by the end of 12 months after a previous remission. Renal activity evaluated by BILAG (British Isles Lupus Assessment Group) scores significantly declined after MSC treatment, in parallel with the obvious amelioration of renal function. Glomerular filtration rate (GFR) improved significantly 12 months after. Total disease activity evaluated by SLEDAI scores also decreased after treatment. Additionally, the doses of concomitant prednisone and immunosuppressive drugs were tapered. No transplantation-related adverse event was observed. They concluded that allogeneic MSC treatment resulted in renal remission for active LN patients within 12-month visit, confirming its use as a potential therapy for refractory LN.

Woodworth et al. [93] examined whether collective data from Wang et al. [71] provided sufficient evidence for the feasibility, safety, dose rationale, and potential efficacy of UC-MSCs to conduct a randomized controlled trial in treatment-refractory SLE nephritis. They observed that results, though confounded by variable baseline prednisone and immuno-suppressive treatment, appear to indicate near term response rates of approximately 50%, which are comparable to those seen with hematopoietic stem cell transplantation but with less morbidity and mortality. They also noticed that apparently, conditioning pre-MSC dosing is not required, although this aspect of the treatment had not been studied in a controlled manner [93].

Another group performed an interesting combination therapy with HSCs and MSCs for life threatening organ involvement involving SLE patient refractory to cyclophosphamide. After being pretreated with CYC, Fudarabine and antithymocyte globulin, the patient was transplanted with autologous CD34+ HSCs and MSCs by intravenous infusion. Hematopoietic regeneration was observed on day 12 thereafter. After HSC and MSC transplantation, the patient's clinical symptoms caused by SLE were remitted, and the SLEDAI score decreased. One more time CD4 + CD25 + FoxP3+ Treg cells were found to be increased in peripheral blood mononuclear cells (PBMCs) after transplantation. This study was important to show that combined transplantation of HSCs and MSCs may reset the adaptive immune system to re-establish self-tolerance in SLE. A 36-month follow-up showed that the clinical symptoms remained in remission for the index patient [94].

A randomized double blind placebo control trial was reported by **Deng et al.** [84] that assessed the efficacy of human umbilical cord-derived mesenchymal stem cell (hUC-MSC) for the treatment of lupus nephritis (LN) among 18 patients with WHO class III or IV LN. Patients were randomly assigned to hUC-MSC (dose 2×10^8 cells) or placebo. All patients received standard immunosuppressive treatment, which consisted of intravenous methylprednisolone and cyclophosphamide, followed by maintenance oral prednisolone and mycophenolate mofetil. Initial 11 patients enrolled to the study received hUC-MSC concurrently with the intravenous methylprednisolone and CYP induction therapy, and for the 12th to 18th patients enrolled, the hUC-MSC were administered together with the intravenous methylprednisolone only and intravenous CYP was delayed to 4 weeks later. In result, similar proportion of patients on hUC-MSC and placebo achieved complete remission. Improvements in serum albumin, complement, renal function, SLEDAI and BILAG scores were similar in both groups. The trial was abandoned after 18 patients were enrolled when it had become obvious it would not demonstrate a positive treatment effect. They concluded that hUC-MSC has no apparent additional effect over and above standard immunosuppression [84].

A pilot study investigated the effect of MSCs on soluble human leukocyte antigen G (s HLA-G) levels 24 hours and 30 days after MSC injection (UC) and reported a negative correlation between the HLA-G levels and clinical SLE activity scores [85]. The levels of s HLA-G were lower in patients with renal involvement than without it.

An open label phase II trial the following year reported safety and long-term efficacy of UC MSCs in severe SLE. Wang et al. [86] reported a long-term follow-up study of allogeneic bone marrow and/or umbilical cord MSC transplantation (MSCT) in severe and drug-refractory systemic lupus erythematosus (SLE) patients. Eighty-one patients were enrolled, and the 5-year overall survival rate was 84% (68/81) after MSCT. At 5-year follow-up, 27% of patients (22/81) were in complete clinical remission and another 7% (6/81) were in partial clinical remission, with a 5-year disease remission rate of 34% (28/81). In total, 37 patients had achieved clinical remission and then 9 patients subsequently relapsed, with 5-year overall rate of relapse of 24% (9/37). SLEDAI scores, serum albumin, complement C3, peripheral white blood cell, and platelet numbers, as well as proteinuria levels, continued to improve during the follow-up. Their results demonstrated that allogeneic MSC treatment is safe and resulted in long-term clinical remission in SLE patients.

Barbado et al. [87] infused three SLE patients with MSCs who were diagnosed with class IV nephritis by kidney biopsies. MSCs were allogeneic MSCs from healthy donors. Total of ninety million cells were infused intravenously into each patient during high and very high activity disease. Patient 1 was treated with cyclophosphamide, azathioprine, methotrexate, mycophenolate and cyclosporine, patient 2 was treated with cyclophosphamide, mycophenolate, rituximab and patient 3 was treated with cyclophosphamide and mycophenolate before MSC treatment. Then, follow-up was performed after 9 months. Proteinuria levels improved significantly during the 1st month and then continued to be sustained in normal levels. Clinical outcome scores such as SLEDAI was perfect for 2 patients while the third SLE patient only had a partial response and the patient could reduce the dose of her current therapies down to 50–60%. Follow up stopped after 9 months SLEDAI scores revealed early, durable, and substantial remissions that were complete for two patients and partial for the third patient and that permitted medication doses to be reduced 50–90%.

In 2019 using slightly older patient population with severe SLE (SLEDAI score > =8), Wen et al. [88] also reported efficacy of allogeneic bone marrow and umbilical cord MSC treatment over one year of follow up in those patients that did not have any baseline arthritis or use of cyclophosphamide of hydroxychloroquine in 2019. Same year Yuan et al. [95] attempted to explore the immunoregulatory mechanism of MSC treatments in SLE patients. They showed that number of peripheral tolerogenic CD1c+ dendritic cells and levels of serum FLT3L are significantly decreased in severely affected SLE patients especially with lupus nephritis. UC-MSC treatment however tapered the FLT3L and inhibited the apoptosis of tolerogenic CD1c + DCs. It is suggested that MSCs carry FLT3L that binds the FLT3 on CD1c + DCs and enhance their ability to proliferate and stops them from being apoptotic [95]. CD1c + DCs in human peripheral blood and in lymphoid and non-lymphoid tissues. CD1c + DCs have been previously reported to play important immune regulatory work such as secreting cytokines when exposed to (poly I:C), LPS or others and regulate the activity of many immune cells such as T regulatory cells and interferon secreting cells [96, 97]. Interferon gamma-FLT3L-FLT3 axis is one of many mechanisms that MSCs are regulating and its implications in treatment of SLE has been recently recognized. Tregs were shown to respond well to allogeneic MSC treatment in several studies. Furthermore, Chen et al. previously have shown that serum HLA-G levels correlated with the levels of Tregs after treatment with allogeneic umbilical cell derived MSCs [85].

Latest report when this chapter was being prepared was by Zhou et al. Zhou et al. [81] did a meta-analysis aiming at assessing whether MSCs can become a new treatment for SLE with good efficacy and safety. Ten studies fulfilled the inclusion criteria and were eligible for this meta-analysis, which comprised 8 prospective or retrospective case series and four randomized controlled trails (RCTs) studies. In the RCT, the results indicated that the MSC group had lower proteinuria than the control group at 3 months and 6 months and the MSC group displayed a lower SLEDAI than the control group at 2 months and 6 months. Furthermore, the MSC group showed a lower rate of adverse events than the control group (OR = 0:26, 95% CI: 0.07, 0.89, P = 0:03). In the case series trials, the results indicated that the MSC group had lower proteinuria at 1 month, 2 months, 3 months, 4 months, 6 months, and 12 months. They concluded that MSCs might be a promising therapeutic agent for patients with SLE. However, they suggested that more studies with longer-term end points and larger sample sizes should be designed and conducted to identify additional and robust patient-centered outcomes in the future [81].

6. Summary/conclusions

The clinical outcome parameters and the kind and amount of MSCs used in the clinical trials we reviewed in this chapter are variable. Most important difference of MSCs used in the clinical trials is whether they are autologous, extracted from the patient's own tissue or allogeneic extracted from health donors. When we reviewed the clinical trials using autologous MSCs trials treating SLE we observed that autologous MSCs did not show much efficacy while allogeneic MSCs regardless of their origins seem to be showing consistently better efficacy in most trials (**Table 1**). The reason for lack of efficacy in autologous use of MSCs is most probably due to their intrinsic abnormalities, and their inability to function at their best capacity. Autologous MSCs may not be functioning due their previous exposure the inflammatory micro environment in SLE or due to their genetic predisposition [79].

Allogeneic mesenchymal stem cell treatment has been shown to be efficacious in the treatment of various systemic lupus erythematosus activity, mainly in refractory lupus nephritis. Allogeneic MSCs, at 1 x 10^6/kg seems to be efficacious but the results are not as homogeneous as expected from clinical trials and FDA approval for MSCs use in rheumatologic diseases have been challenging. Heterogeneous results could be due to the heterogenous disease manifestations among patients enrolled to the clinical trials. In addition, although there are plenty of MSC trial reports that shows evidence for MSCs efficacy in SLE, randomized prospective controlled trials using MSCs are still missing.

In addition, the tissue source of donor MSCs shows remarkable variability, while some investigators believe in the superior anti-inflammatory effects of audiogenic MSCs other disagree and suggest umbilical cord MSCs immune modulatory efficacies. Since future MSC clinical trials and MSC therapies will be dependent on the availability of the donor tissue, technologic advancement to optimize the MSCs that can be easily obtained such as adipogenic tissue or peripheral blood must be prioritized.

Most MSC products used in clinical trials still lack a clear product definition, how they are selected, and application protocols. It is possible that the dose, route and frequency of the cell product protocol used in a clinical trial may not be universally applicable. Furthermore, due to the ever-thriving knowledge about MSCs functions we are yet to establish clear outcome criteria for testing MSC efficacy and safety.

Most MSC clinical trials have the inclusion criteria to enroll patients with severe disease activity and criteria of failure of currently available treatments. Therefore, there might be already irreversible and secondary tissue damage and MSCs may not be able to reverse this outcome when used in the late phase of the organ damage. If MSCs can be given in an earlier stage of disease their efficacy might be a lot better.

In summary, as you would see from the list of clinical trials and their outcomes (**Table 1**) discussed in this chapter the investigators that take roles in MSC clinical trials are not only struggling with the source of MSCs and optimization of efficacy they are also facing very complex regulatory issues. The variable sources of stem cells, cumbersome manufacturing processes are further complicating design of clinical trials. Further studies assessing the efficacy of MSC treatments needs to be performed.

Author details

Hulya Bukulmez* and Gurinder Kumar
Department of Pediatrics, Division of Pediatric Rheumatology, MetroHealth Medical Center, Case Western Reserve University, Cleveland, Ohio, USA

*Address all correspondence to: hxb38@case.edu

References

[1] Maroz N and Segal MS. Lupus nephritis and end-stage kidney disease. *Am J Med Sci* 2013; 346: 319-323. 2013/02/02. DOI: 10.1097/MAJ.0b013e31827f4ee3.

[2] Mavragani CP and Moutsopoulos HM. Sjogren's syndrome: Old and new therapeutic targets. *J Autoimmun* 2020; 110: 102364. 2019/12/14. DOI: 10.1016/j.jaut.2019.102364.

[3] Ball LM, Egeler RM and Party EPW. Acute GvHD: pathogenesis and classification. *Bone Marrow Transplant* 2008; 41 Suppl 2: S58-64. 2008/07/24. DOI: 10.1038/bmt.2008.56.

[4] Bawazier LA. Current and Emerging Therapy on Lupus Nephritis. *Acta Med Indones* 2017; 49: 369-377. 2018/01/20.

[5] Raja TW, Veeramuthu D, Savarimuthu I, et al. Current Trends in the Treatment of Systemic Lupus Erythematosus. *Curr Pharm Des* 2020; 26: 2602-2609. 2020/02/19. DOI: 10.2174/1381612826666200211122633.

[6] Hanly JG, Kozora E, Beyea SD, et al. Review: Nervous System Disease in Systemic Lupus Erythematosus: Current Status and Future Directions. *Arthritis Rheumatol* 2019; 71: 33-42. 2018/06/22. DOI: 10.1002/art.40591.

[7] Adam Z, Sokwala A, Shah J, et al. A delay in diagnosis: thrombotic thrombocytopenia purpura occurring in systemic lupus erythematous. *Pan Afr Med J* 2019; 34: 103. 2020/01/15. DOI: 10.11604/pamj.2019.34.103.20524.

[8] Safiri S, Kolahi AA, Cross M, et al. Global, regional, and national burden of other musculoskeletal disorders 1990-2017: results from the Global Burden of Disease Study 2017. *Rheumatology (Oxford)* 2020 2020/08/26. DOI: 10.1093/rheumatology/keaa315.

[9] Tanaka Y, O'Neill S, Li M, et al. Systemic Lupus Erythematosus: Targeted literature review of the epidemiology, current treatment and disease burden in the Asia Pacific region. *Arthritis Care Res (Hoboken)* 2020 2020/08/26. DOI: 10.1002/acr.24431.

[10] McCormick N, Marra CA, Sadatsafavi M, et al. Socioeconomic status at diagnosis influences the incremental direct medical costs of systemic lupus erythematosus: A longitudinal population-based study. *Semin Arthritis Rheum* 2020; 50: 77-83. 2019/07/31. DOI: 10.1016/j.semarthrit.2019.06.010.

[11] Bezalel S, Guri KM, Elbirt D, et al. Type I interferon signature in systemic lupus erythematosus. *Isr Med Assoc J* 2014; 16: 246-249. 2014/05/20.

[12] Dema B and Charles N. Advances in mechanisms of systemic lupus erythematosus. *Discov Med* 2014; 17: 247-255. 2014/06/03.

[13] Torell F, Eketjall S, Idborg H, et al. Cytokine Profiles in Autoantibody Defined Subgroups of Systemic Lupus Erythematosus. *J Proteome Res* 2019; 18: 1208-1217. 2019/02/12. DOI: 10.1021/acs.jproteome.8b00811.

[14] Hayashi T. Therapeutic strategies for SLE involving cytokines: mechanism-oriented therapies especially IFN-gamma targeting gene therapy. *J Biomed Biotechnol* 2010; 2010 2010/09/10. DOI: 10.1155/2010/461641.

[15] O'Neill S and Cervera R. Systemic lupus erythematosus. *Best Pract Res Clin Rheumatol* 2010; 24: 841-855. 2011/06/15. DOI: 10.1016/j.berh.2010.10.006.

[16] Trucci VM, Salum FG, Figueiredo MA, et al. Interrelationship

of dendritic cells, type 1 interferon system, regulatory T cells and toll-like receptors and their role in lichen planus and lupus erythematosus -- a literature review. *Arch Oral Biol* 2013; 58: 1532-1540. 2013/07/13. DOI: 10.1016/j.archoralbio.2013.06.016.

[17] Larkin J, 3rd, Ahmed CM, Wilson TD, et al. Regulation of interferon gamma signaling by suppressors of cytokine signaling and regulatory T cells. *Front Immunol* 2013; 4: 469. 2014/01/07. DOI: 10.3389/fimmu.2013.00469.

[18] Talaat RM, Mohamed SF, Bassyouni IH, et al. Th1/Th2/Th17/Treg cytokine imbalance in systemic lupus erythematosus (SLE) patients: Correlation with disease activity. *Cytokine* 2015; 72: 146-153. 2015/02/04. DOI: 10.1016/j.cyto.2014.12.027.

[19] Liu Y, Liao J, Zhao M, et al. Increased expression of TLR2 in CD4(+) T cells from SLE patients enhances immune reactivity and promotes IL-17 expression through histone modifications. *Eur J Immunol* 2015; 45: 2683-2693. 2015/06/17. DOI: 10.1002/eji.201445219.

[20] Mizui M, Koga T, Lieberman LA, et al. IL-2 protects lupus-prone mice from multiple end-organ damage by limiting CD4-CD8- IL-17-producing T cells. *J Immunol* 2014; 193: 2168-2177. 2014/07/27. DOI: 10.4049/jimmunol.1400977.

[21] Rafael-Vidal C, Perez N, Altabas I, et al. Blocking IL-17: A Promising Strategy in the Treatment of Systemic Rheumatic Diseases. *Int J Mol Sci* 2020; 21 2020/10/01. DOI: 10.3390/ijms21197100.

[22] Mohammadi S, Sedighi S and Memarian A. IL-17 is Aberrantly Overexpressed Among Under-treatment Systemic Lupus Erythematosus Patients. *Iran J Pathol* 2019; 14: 236-242. 2019/10/05. DOI: 10.30699/ijp.2019.94878.1934.

[23] Li QZ, Zhou J, Lian Y, et al. Interferon signature gene expression is correlated with autoantibody profiles in patients with incomplete lupus syndromes. *Clin Exp Immunol*; 159: 281-291. 2009/12/09. DOI: CEI4057 [pii] 10.1111/j.1365-2249.2009.04057.x.

[24] Hahn BH, Anderson M, Le E, et al. Anti-DNA Ig peptides promote Treg cell activity in systemic lupus erythematosus patients. *Arthritis Rheum* 2008; 58: 2488-2497. 2008/08/01. DOI: 10.1002/art.23609.

[25] Lee PY and Reeves WH. Type I interferon as a target of treatment in SLE. *Endocr Metab Immune Disord Drug Targets* 2006; 6: 323-330. 2007/01/12.

[26] Zhuang H, Kosboth M, Lee P, et al. Lupus-like disease and high interferon levels corresponding to trisomy of the type I interferon cluster on chromosome 9p. *Arthritis Rheum* 2006; 54: 1573-1579. 2006/04/29. DOI: 10.1002/art.21800.

[27] Mangini AJ, Lafyatis R and Van Seventer JM. Type I interferons inhibition of inflammatory T helper cell responses in systemic lupus erythematosus. *Ann N Y Acad Sci* 2007; 1108: 11-23. 2007/09/26. DOI: 10.1196/annals.1422.002.

[28] Sozzani S, Bosisio D, Scarsi M, et al. Type I interferons in systemic autoimmunity. *Autoimmunity* 2010; 43: 196-203. 2010/03/20. DOI: 10.3109/08916930903510872.

[29] Ronnblom L. The importance of the type I interferon system in autoimmunity. *Clin Exp Rheumatol* 2016; 34: 21-24. 2016/09/03.

[30] Yan B, Ye S, Chen G, et al. Dysfunctional CD4+,CD25+ regulatory T cells in untreated active systemic lupus erythematosus secondary to interferon-alpha-producing antigen-presenting cells. *Arthritis Rheum* 2008; 58: 801-812. 2008/03/04. DOI: 10.1002/art.23268.

[31] Ferreira RC, Castro Dopico X, Oliveira JJ, et al. Chronic Immune Activation in Systemic Lupus Erythematosus and the Autoimmune PTPN22 Trp(620) Risk Allele Drive the Expansion of FOXP3(+) Regulatory T Cells and PD-1 Expression. *Front Immunol* 2019; 10: 2606. 2019/11/30. DOI: 10.3389/fimmu.2019.02606.

[32] Kailashiya V, Singh U, Rana R, et al. Regulatory T Cells and Their Association with Serum Markers and Symptoms in Systemic Lupus Erythematosus and Rheumatoid Arthritis. *Immunol Invest* 2019; 48: 64-78. 2018/10/17. DOI: 10.1080/08820139.2018.1527852.

[33] Dall'Era M, Pauli ML, Remedios K, et al. Adoptive Treg Cell Therapy in a Patient With Systemic Lupus Erythematosus. *Arthritis Rheumatol* 2019; 71: 431-440. 2018/10/03. DOI: 10.1002/art.40737.

[34] Ptacek T, Li X, Kelley JM, et al. Copy number variants in genetic susceptibility and severity of systemic lupus erythematosus. *Cytogenet Genome Res* 2008; 123: 142-147. 2008/01/01. DOI: 000184701 [pii]10.1159/000184701.

[35] Levine AB and Erkan D. Clinical assessment and management of cytopenias in lupus patients. Curr Rheumatol Rep 2011; 13: 291-299. DOI: 10.1007/s11926-011-0179-5.

[36] Tsokos GC, Lo MS, Costa Reis P, et al. New insights into the immunopathogenesis of systemic lupus erythematosus. *Nat Rev Rheumatol* 2016; 12: 716-730. 2016/11/23. DOI: 10.1038/nrrheum.2016.186.

[37] Zhang L, Bertucci AM, Ramsey-Goldman R, et al. Regulatory T cell (Treg) subsets return in patients with refractory lupus following stem cell transplantation, and TGF-beta-producing CD8+ Treg cells are associated with immunological remission of lupus. *J Immunol* 2009; 183: 6346-6358. 2009/10/21. DOI: 10.4049/jimmunol.0901773.

[38] Jaiswal N, Haynesworth SE, Caplan AI, et al. Osteogenic differentiation of purified, culture-expanded human mesenchymal stem cells in vitro. *J Cell Biochem* 1997; 64: 295-312. 1997/02/01. DOI: 10.1002/(SICI)1097-4644(199702)64:2<295::AID-JCB12>3.0.CO;2-I [pii].

[39] Lennon DP, Schluchter MD and Caplan AI. The effect of extended first passage culture on the proliferation and differentiation of human marrow-derived mesenchymal stem cells. *Stem Cells Transl Med* 2012; 1: 279-288. 2012/12/01. DOI: 10.5966/sctm.2011-0011.

[40] Somoza RA, Welter JF, Correa D, et al. Chondrogenic differentiation of mesenchymal stem cells: challenges and unfulfilled expectations. *Tissue Eng Part B Rev* 2014; 20: 596-608. 2014/04/23. DOI: 10.1089/ten.TEB.2013.0771.

[41] Lee Z, Dennis J, Alsberg E, et al. Imaging stem cell differentiation for cell-based tissue repair. *Methods Enzymol* 2012; 506: 247-263. 2012/02/22. DOI: 10.1016/B978-0-12-391856-7.00037-8.

[42] Li R, Liang L, Dou Y, et al. Mechanical stretch inhibits mesenchymal stem cell adipogenic differentiation through TGFbeta1/Smad2 signaling. J Biomech 2015; 48: 3665-3671. DOI: 10.1016/j.jbiomech.2015.08.013.

[43] Bourin P, Bunnell BA, Casteilla L, et al. Stromal cells from the adipose tissue-derived stromal vascular fraction and culture expanded adipose tissue-derived stromal/stem cells: a joint statement of the International Federation for Adipose Therapeutics and Science (IFATS) and the

International Society for Cellular Therapy (ISCT). *Cytotherapy* 2013; 15: 641-648. 2013/04/11. DOI: 10.1016/j.jcyt.2013.02.006.

[44] Tyndall A and Uccelli A. Multipotent mesenchymal stromal cells for autoimmune diseases: teaching new dogs old tricks. *Bone Marrow Transplant* 2009; 43: 821-828. 2009/03/25. DOI: 10.1038/bmt.2009.63.

[45] Dominici M, Le Blanc K, Mueller I, et al. Minimal criteria for defining multipotent mesenchymal stromal cells. The International Society for Cellular Therapy position statement. *Cytotherapy* 2006; 8: 315-317. 2006/08/23. DOI: 10.1080/14653240600855905.

[46] Stacey GN, Andrews PW, Barbaric I, et al. Stem cell culture conditions and stability: a joint workshop of the PluriMes Consortium and Pluripotent Stem Cell Platform. *Regen Med* 2019; 14: 243-255. 2019/04/03. DOI: 10.2217/rme-2019-0001.

[47] Duffy MM, McNicholas BA, Monaghan DA, et al. Mesenchymal stem cells and a vitamin D receptor agonist additively suppress T helper 17 cells and the related inflammatory response in the kidney. *Am J Physiol Renal Physiol* 2014; 307: F1412-1426. 2014/10/24. DOI: 10.1152/ajprenal.00024.2014.

[48] Darlington PJ, Boivin MN, Renoux C, et al. Reciprocal Th1 and Th17 regulation by mesenchymal stem cells: Implication for multiple sclerosis. *Ann Neurol* 2010/07/28. DOI: 10.1002/ana.22065.

[49] Leyendecker A, Jr., Pinheiro CCG, Amano MT, et al. The Use of Human Mesenchymal Stem Cells as Therapeutic Agents for the in vivo Treatment of Immune-Related Diseases: A Systematic Review. *Front Immunol* 2018; 9: 2056. 2018/09/27. DOI: 10.3389/fimmu.2018.02056.

[50] Bai L, Lennon DP, Eaton V, et al. Human bone marrow-derived mesenchymal stem cells induce Th2-polarized immune response and promote endogenous repair in animal models of multiple sclerosis. *Glia* 2009; 57: 1192-1203. 2009/02/05. DOI: 10.1002/glia.20841.

[51] Wang D, Huang S, Yuan X, et al. The regulation of the Treg/Th17 balance by mesenchymal stem cells in human systemic lupus erythematosus. *Cell Mol Immunol* 2017; 14: 423-431. 2015/10/06. DOI: 10.1038/cmi.2015.89.

[52] Ghannam S, Pene J, Moquet-Torcy G, et al. Mesenchymal stem cells inhibit human Th17 cell differentiation and function and induce a T regulatory cell phenotype. *J Immunol* 2010; 185: 302-312. 2010/06/01. DOI: 10.4049/jimmunol.0902007.

[53] Pianta S, Bonassi Signoroni P, Muradore I, et al. Amniotic membrane mesenchymal cells-derived factors skew T cell polarization toward Treg and downregulate Th1 and Th17 cells subsets. *Stem Cell Rev Rep* 2015; 11: 394-407. 2014/10/29. DOI: 10.1007/s12015-014-9558-4.

[54] Zeng SL, Wang LH, Li P, et al. Mesenchymal stem cells abrogate experimental asthma by altering dendritic cell function. Mol Med Rep 2015; 12: 2511-2520. DOI: 10.3892/mmr.2015.3706.

[55] Liang J and Sun L. Mesenchymal stem cells transplantation for systemic lupus erythematosus. *Int J Rheum Dis* 2015; 18: 164-171. 2015/01/23. DOI: 10.1111/1756-185X.12531.

[56] De Miguel MP, Fuentes-Julian S, Blazquez-Martinez A, et al. Immunosuppressive properties of mesenchymal stem cells: advances and applications. *Curr Mol Med* 2012; 12: 574-591. 2012/04/21.

[57] Gao C, Wang X, Lu J, et al. Mesenchymal stem cells transfected with sFgl2 inhibit the acute rejection of heart transplantation in mice by regulating macrophage activation. *Stem Cell Res Ther* 2020; 11: 241. 2020/06/20. DOI: 10.1186/s13287-020-01752-1.

[58] Cho DI, Kim MR, Jeong HY, et al. Mesenchymal stem cells reciprocally regulate the M1/M2 balance in mouse bone marrow-derived macrophages. *Exp Mol Med* 2014; 46: e70. 2014/01/11. DOI: 10.1038/emm.2013.135.

[59] Geng Y, Zhang L, Fu B, et al. Mesenchymal stem cells ameliorate rhabdomyolysis-induced acute kidney injury via the activation of M2 macrophages. *Stem Cell Res Ther* 2014; 5: 80. 2014/06/26. DOI: 10.1186/scrt469.

[60] Song T, Eirin A, Zhu X, et al. Mesenchymal Stem Cell-Derived Extracellular Vesicles Induce Regulatory T Cells to Ameliorate Chronic Kidney Injury. *Hypertension* 2020; 75: 1223-1232. 2020/04/01. DOI: 10.1161/HYPERTENSIONAHA.119.14546.

[61] Poltavtsev AM, Poltavtseva RA, Yushina MN, et al. Cytokine Production in Mixed Cultures of Mesenchymal Stromal Cells from Wharton's Jelly and Peripheral Blood Lymphocytes. *Bull Exp Biol Med* 2017; 163: 169-175. 2017/06/06. DOI: 10.1007/s10517-017-3759-1.

[62] Chen HW, Chen HY, Wang LT, et al. Mesenchymal stem cells tune the development of monocyte-derived dendritic cells toward a myeloid-derived suppressive phenotype through growth-regulated oncogene chemokines. *J Immunol* 2013; 190: 5065-5077. 2013/04/17. DOI: 10.4049/jimmunol.1202775.

[63] Cui R, Rekasi H, Hepner-Schefczyk M, et al. Human mesenchymal stromal/stem cells acquire immunostimulatory capacity upon cross-talk with natural killer cells and might improve the NK cell function of immunocompromised patients. *Stem Cell Res Ther* 2016; 7: 88. 2016/07/09. DOI: 10.1186/s13287-016-0353-9.

[64] Wang D, Feng X, Lu L, et al. A CD8 T cell/indoleamine 2,3-dioxygenase axis is required for mesenchymal stem cell suppression of human systemic lupus erythematosus. *Arthritis Rheumatol* 2014; 66: 2234-2245. 2014/04/24. DOI: 10.1002/art.38674.

[65] Cassano JM, Schnabel LV, Goodale MB, et al. The immunomodulatory function of equine MSCs is enhanced by priming through an inflammatory microenvironment or TLR3 ligand. Vet Immunol Immunopathol 2018; 195: 33-39. DOI: 10.1016/j.vetimm.2017.10.003.

[66] da Silva Meirelles L, Caplan AI and Nardi NB. In search of the in vivo identity of mesenchymal stem cells. *Stem Cells* 2008; 26: 2287-2299. 2008/06/21. DOI: 10.1634/stemcells.2007-1122.

[67] da Silva Meirelles L, Sand TT, Harman RJ, et al. MSC frequency correlates with blood vessel density in equine adipose tissue. *Tissue Eng Part A* 2009; 15: 221-229. 2008/10/14. DOI: 10.1089/ten.tea.2008.0103.

[68] Spitzer TL, Rojas A, Zelenko Z, et al. Perivascular human endometrial mesenchymal stem cells express pathways relevant to self-renewal, lineage specification, and functional phenotype. *Biol Reprod* 2012; 86: 58. 2011/11/15. DOI: 10.1095/biolreprod.111.095885.

[69] Caplan AI. New era of cell-based orthopedic therapies. *Tissue Eng Part B Rev* 2009; 15: 195-200. 2009/02/21. DOI: 10.1089/ten.TEB.2008.0515.

[70] Rodriguez-Fuentes DE, Fernandez-Garza LE, Samia-Meza JA, et al. Mesenchymal Stem Cells Current

Clinical Applications: A Systematic Review. *Arch Med Res* 2020 2020/09/27. DOI: 10.1016/j.arcmed.2020.08.006.

[71] Wang D, Li J, Zhang Y, et al. Umbilical cord mesenchymal stem cell transplantation in active and refractory systemic lupus erythematosus: a multicenter clinical study. *Arthritis Res Ther* 2014; 16: R79. 2014/03/26. DOI: 10.1186/ar4520.

[72] Gu F, Wang D, Zhang H, et al. Allogeneic mesenchymal stem cell transplantation for lupus nephritis patients refractory to conventional therapy. *Clin Rheumatol* 2014; 33: 1611-1619. 2014/08/15. DOI: 10.1007/s10067-014-2754-4.

[73] Jayne D and Tyndall A. Autologous stem cell transplantation for systemic lupus erythematosus. *Lupus* 2004; 13: 359-365. 2004/07/03. DOI: 10.1191/0961203304lu1027oa.

[74] Jayne D, Passweg J, Marmont A, et al. Autologous stem cell transplantation for systemic lupus erythematosus. *Lupus* 2004; 13: 168-176. 2004/05/04. DOI: 10.1191/0961203304lu525oa.

[75] Burt RK, Traynor A, Statkute L, et al. Nonmyeloablative hematopoietic stem cell transplantation for systemic lupus erythematosus. *JAMA* 2006; 295: 527-535. 2006/02/02. DOI: 10.1001/jama.295.5.527.

[76] Burt RK, Verda L, Oyama Y, et al. Non-myeloablative stem cell transplantation for autoimmune diseases. *Springer Semin Immunopathol* 2004; 26: 57-69. 2004/11/19. DOI: 10.1007/s00281-004-0162-6.

[77] Sun L, Wang D, Liang J, et al. Umbilical cord mesenchymal stem cell transplantation in severe and refractory systemic lupus erythematosus. *Arthritis Rheum* 2010; 62: 2467-2475. 2010/05/28. DOI: 10.1002/art.27548.

[78] Liang J, Zhang H, Hua B, et al. Allogenic mesenchymal stem cells transplantation in refractory systemic lupus erythematosus: a pilot clinical study. *Ann Rheum Dis* 2010; 69: 1423-1429. 2010/07/24. DOI: 10.1136/ard.2009.123463.

[79] Carrion F, Nova E, Ruiz C, et al. Autologous mesenchymal stem cell treatment increased T regulatory cells with no effect on disease activity in two systemic lupus erythematosus patients. *Lupus* 2010; 19: 317-322. 2009/11/19. DOI: 10.1177/0961203309348983.

[80] Shi D, Wang D, Li X, Zhang H, Che N, Lu Z, et al. Allogeneic transplantation of umbilical cord-derived mesenchymal stem cells for diffuse alveolar hemorrhage in systemic lupus erythematosus. Clin Rheumatol. 2012;31(5):841-846. doi: 10.1007/s10067-012-1943-2.

[81] Zhou T, Li HY, Liao C, et al. Clinical Efficacy and Safety of Mesenchymal Stem Cells for Systemic Lupus Erythematosus. *Stem Cells Int* 2020; 2020: 6518508. 2020/04/24. DOI: 10.1155/2020/6518508.

[82] Li X, Wang D, Liang J, Zhang H, Sun L. Mesenchymal SCT ameliorates refractory cytopenia in patients with systemic lupus erythematosus. Bone Marrow Transplant. 2013;48(4):544-550. doi: 10.1038/bmt.2012.184.

[83] Wang D, Zhang H, Liang J, et al. Allogeneic mesenchymal stem cell transplantation in severe and refractory systemic lupus erythematosus: 4 years of experience. *Cell Transplant* 2013; 22: 2267-2277. 2014/01/07. DOI: 10.3727/096368911X582769c.

[84] Deng D, Zhang P, Guo Y, et al. A randomised double-blind, placebo-controlled trial of allogeneic umbilical cord-derived mesenchymal stem cell for lupus nephritis. *Ann Rheum Dis* 2017; 76: 1436-1439. 2017/05/10. DOI: 10.1136/annrheumdis-2017-211073.

[85] Chen C, Liang J, Yao G, et al. Mesenchymal stem cells upregulate Treg cells via sHLA-G in SLE patients. *Int Immunopharmacol* 2017; 44: 234-241. 2017/01/28. DOI: 10.1016/j.intimp.2017.01.024.

[86] Wang D, Zhang H, Liang J, et al. A Long-Term Follow-Up Study of Allogeneic Mesenchymal Stem/Stromal Cell Transplantation in Patients with Drug-Resistant Systemic Lupus Erythematosus. *Stem Cell Reports* 2018; 10: 933-941. 2018/02/27. DOI: 10.1016/j.stemcr.2018.01.029.

[87] Barbado J, Tabera S, Sanchez A, et al. Therapeutic potential of allogeneic mesenchymal stromal cells transplantation for lupus nephritis. *Lupus* 2018; 27: 2161-2165. 2018/10/07. DOI: 10.1177/0961203318804922.

[88] Wen L, Labopin M, Badoglio M, et al. Prognostic Factors for Clinical Response in Systemic Lupus Erythematosus Patients Treated by Allogeneic Mesenchymal Stem Cells. *Stem Cells Int* 2019; 2019: 7061408. 2019/06/14. DOI: 10.1155/2019/7061408.

[89] Le Blanc K, Rasmusson I, Sundberg B, et al. Treatment of severe acute graft-versus-host disease with third party haploidentical mesenchymal stem cells. *Lancet* 2004; 363: 1439-1441. 2004/05/04. DOI: 10.1016/S0140-6736(04)16104-7.

[90] Nie Y, Lau CS, Lie AK, et al. Defective phenotype of mesenchymal stem cells in patients with systemic lupus erythematosus. *Lupus* 2010/02/02. DOI: 0961203310361482 [pii]10.1177/0961203310361482.

[91] Sui W, Hou X, Che W, et al. Hematopoietic and mesenchymal stem cell transplantation for severe and refractory systemic lupus erythematosus. *Clin Immunol* 2013; 148: 186-197. 2013/06/19. DOI: 10.1016/j.clim.2013.05.014.

[92] Belimumab. No tangible efficacy but a risk of immunosuppression. Prescrire Int 2013; 22: 149.

[93] Woodworth TG and Furst DE. Safety and feasibility of umbilical cord mesenchymal stem cells in treatment-refractory systemic lupus erythematosus nephritis: time for a double-blind placebo-controlled trial to determine efficacy. *Arthritis Res Ther* 2014; 16: 113. 2014/08/29. DOI: 10.1186/ar4677.

[94] Wang Q, Qian S, Li J, et al. Combined transplantation of autologous hematopoietic stem cells and allogenic mesenchymal stem cells increases T regulatory cells in systemic lupus erythematosus with refractory lupus nephritis and leukopenia. *Lupus* 2015; 24: 1221-1226. 2015/04/29. DOI: 10.1177/0961203315583541.

[95] Yuan X, Qin X, Wang D, et al. Mesenchymal stem cell therapy induces FLT3L and CD1c(+) dendritic cells in systemic lupus erythematosus patients. *Nat Commun* 2019; 10: 2498. 2019/06/09. DOI: 10.1038/s41467-019-10491-8.

[96] Liu J and Cao X. Regulatory dendritic cells in autoimmunity: A comprehensive review. *J Autoimmun* 2015; 63: 1-12. 2015/08/10. DOI: 10.1016/j.jaut.2015.07.011.

[97] Bamboat ZM, Stableford JA, Plitas G, et al. Human liver dendritic cells promote T cell hyporesponsiveness. *J Immunol* 2009; 182: 1901-1911. 2009/02/10. DOI: 10.4049/jimmunol.0803404.